2025

Wood Snake Year
FENG SHUI
AND CHINESE ASTROLOGY
PLANNER

MICHELE CASTLE

Welcome to the energies of the Wood Snake in 2025! This year is guided by the graceful and enigmatic Wood Snake, a symbol of wisdom, intuition, and transformation. Snakes are known for their calm, reflective nature and keen perception, though they can sometimes be secretive and reserved. Despite this, their allure is captivating, and they possess an innate ability to navigate life's complexities with grace and insight.

The Wood Snake of 2025, with its unique blend of wisdom, intuition, and transformation, embodies these traits distinctively from other years. It acts as a quiet yet powerful force of change, exuding subtle sophistication and strategic thinking. These quintessential Snake characteristics will be deeply woven into the year's energy, shaping the experiences and opportunities ahead.

In 2025, the Snake aligns with the Wood element, symbolising a time for thoughtful planning, patience, and the cultivation of long-term growth and prosperity. The wood element, as the fuel for Fire, also ignites passion, creativity, and the birth of new ideas. This combination makes 2025 a year for strategic innovation and deeper exploration, with the Wood element playing a pivotal role in shaping these opportunities.

The 2025 Astrology & Feng Shui diary provides daily insights into your health, relationships, and business opportunities, offering valuable guidance from Chinese Astrology, Flying Star, and the Bagua School. It's a practical tool to help you navigate the year with confidence and control.

Embrace the transformations and energies that 2025 brings:

- · A year of introspection and subtle progress.
- · A time for wisdom and intuition.
- · A period marked by strategic movement and quiet determination.
- · Anticipate profound shifts and insightful revelations.

While Feng Shui doesn't offer magical solutions, understanding and wisely placing symbolic cures can help minimise challenges during these transformative times. By embracing the profound science of Feng Shui, you can adapt more effectively to the changing energies in your environment, home, and the world. Feng Shui, meaning "wind and water," reflects the essence of life's energy and fluidity, grounding you in a realistic approach to change.

May 2025 bring health, harmony, and prosperity as you navigate life's flowing waters and shifting winds.

Michele

Published by Complete Feng Shui
Mb: 0421 116 799,
Email: info@completefengshui.com.au
Websites: www.completefengshui.com

Author: Michele Castle
Design copyright @completefengshui
Title: 2025 Feng Shui & Astrology Planner

ISBN: 978-0-6459097-8-4 (Paperback)
ISBN: 978-0-6459097-9-1 (Hardcover)
ISBN: 978-0-6452137-3-7 (EPUB)

October 2024

This Planner has been written to offer insight and planning for daily activities and energies in 2025 from Flying Stars, Bagua, Chinese astrology, and date selection. The author, editor and publisher take no responsibility for the outcome of any information implemented from this Diary.

This planner's information is summarised from the Chinese Thousand Year Calendar and presented as user-friendly to help you enjoy prosperity throughout the year.

Vice President of the Association of Feng Shui Consultants (AFSC)
Platinum member of the Association of Feng Shui Consultants (AFSC)
Recognised Feng Shui training institution by the (AFSC)

facebook@completefengshui   instagram@completefengshui

CONTENTS

Personal details vii

Resolutions for 2025 ix

2025 Year of Wood Dragon 1

Chinese New Year Traditions 3

Auspicious Feng Shui Colours for 2024 5

How to Use the Complete Feng Shui Planner 7

Flying Star Feng Shui 8

Favourable Stars / Unfavourable Stars 9

2025 Afflictions 10

January 6 – February 3 is month of the Ox 12

January Flying Stars 14

January Monthly Chinese Zodiac Overview 16

The Feng Shui of Your Front Door 20

February 4 – March 5 is month of the Tiger 24

February Flying Stars 26

February Monthly Chinese Zodiac Overview 28

March 6 – April 4 is month of the Rabbit 34

March Flying Stars 36

March Monthly Chinese Zodiac Overview 38

April 5 – May 5 is month of the Dragon 44

April Flying Stars 46

April Monthly Chinese Zodiac Overview 48

Feng Shui Principles of the Bedroom 52

May 6 – June 5 is month of the Snake 56

May Flying Stars 58

May Monthly Chinese Zodiac Overview 60

June 6 – July 6 is month of the Horse 66

June Flying Stars 68

June Monthly Chinese Zodiac Overview 70

July 7 – August 7 is month of the Goat..76

July Flying Stars..78

July Monthly Chinese Zodiac Overview..80

August 8 – September 7 is month of the Monkey 86

August Flying Stars 88

August Monthly Chinese Zodiac Overview 90

Ideal Kitchen placement in Feng Shui...94

September 8 – October 7 is month of the Rooster......................................98

September Flying Stars...100

September Monthly Chinese Zodiac Overview..102

Activating Peach Blossom luck for relationship & marriage luck.............106

October 8 – November 6 is month of the Dog 110

October Flying Stars..112

October Monthly Chinese Zodiac Overview...114

November 7 – December 6 is month of the Pig..120

Eight Aspirations Formula...121

November Flying Stars...122

November Monthly Chinese Zodiac Overview...124

December 7 – January 5 is month of the Rat..130

December Flying Stars...132

December Monthly Chinese Zodiac Overview...134

Activating Feng Shui in the Garden..138

Your Kua Number 142

Auspicious and Inauspicious directions based on your Kua Number 147

Calendar 2025...148

Calendar 2026...149

Planner 2025 150

WELCOME

2025 NEW BEGINNINGS

Your Personal Information

Name ....

Date of Birth ....

Time of Birth ....

Animal Sign ....

Address ....

....

....

Telephone No. .... Office No. ....

Mobile No .... Fax No. ....

E-mail address ....

Favorite Websites ....

....

Secret Friend .... Allies ....

Conflict Animal ....

Peach Blossom Animal ....

Self-Element ....

Kua Number ....

Your House Facing Direction ....

Office Direction ....

Best Direction (Sheng Chi) .... Health Direction (Tien Yi) ....

Romance Direction (Nien Yen) .... Personal Growth Direction (Fu Wei)............

Unlucky (Ho Hai) .... Five Ghost (Wu Kwei) ....

Six Killings (Lui Sha) .... Total Loss (Chueh Ming) ....

Resolutions for 2025

....

....

....

....

....

....

....

....

....

....

....

....

....

The Snake symbolises wisdom, transformation, and deep intuition in Chinese mythology. For 2025, the Year of the Wood Snake, the Snake embodies the power of quiet strength, adaptability, and regeneration. Revered for its ability to shed its skin, the Snake represents personal growth, renewal, and the shedding old habits to make way for new beginnings. Linked to protection and spiritual insight, the Snake is believed to guard against misfortune and harmful energies. Its connection to the earth and hidden depths also signifies inner knowledge and harmony with nature. The Snake's mysterious yet wise nature aligns it with the balance of Yin and Yang, while its enduring presence in Chinese culture speaks to longevity and the cyclical nature of life. As a symbol of transformation, protection, and intuitive wisdom, the Snake brings an auspicious blend of subtle power and cultural significance in 2025.

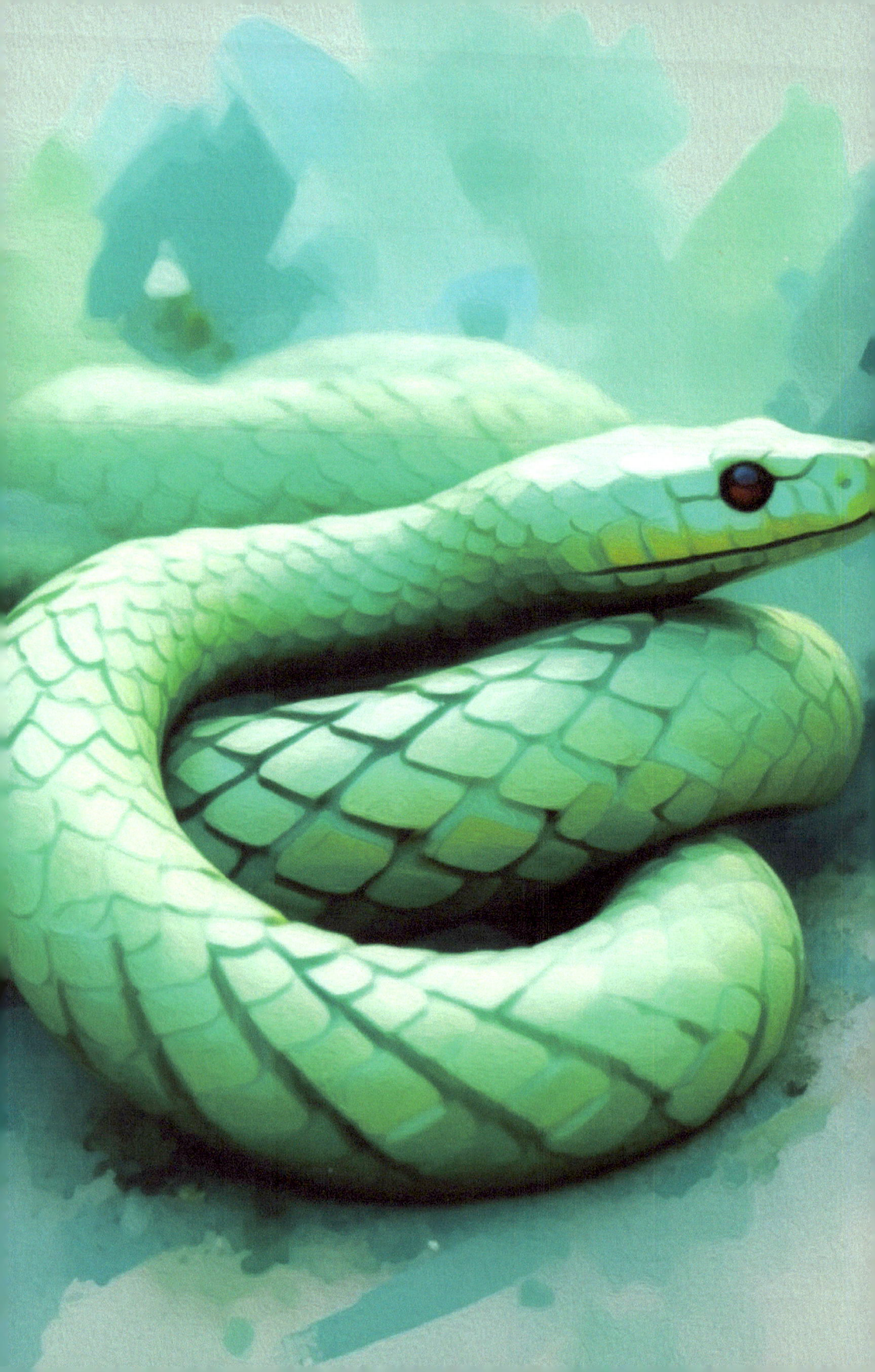

2025 YEAR OF WOOD SNAKE

Subtle yet transformative energies symbolise the Year of the Wood Snake in 2025. Like the delicate but resilient forms of nature it is connected to, this year represents growth, change, and renewal. It thrives with sunlight and water and can withstand strong winds, embodying innovation, adaptability, and silent strength.

The Snake, an emblem of wisdom, spiritual growth, and rejuvenation, holds profound significance in Chinese culture. Known for shedding its skin, the Snake represents rebirth and transformation, reminding us that patience and letting go of the past are essential for new beginnings. In 2025, this message will resonate deeply, encouraging us to embrace change and personal growth amid challenges.

As the sixth sign of the Chinese Zodiac, the Snake is associated with intelligence, grace, and strategic thinking. Those born under this sign are known for their sharp analytical skills and ability to make well-considered decisions. However, in extreme cases, the Snake's influence can lead to over-caution or manipulation to achieve goals. This year, it is essential to balance wisdom with integrity to navigate life's complexities.

Clashing signs in 2025 include the Pig, Monkey, Tiger, and Snake. Those born under these signs may experience movement and change, such as travelling, relocating, or switching careers. In Ba Zi, the Four Pillars of Destiny, these signs are considered 'Travelling Horses.' This term represents dynamic energy that can propel shifts in various areas of life. For individuals affected by these clashes, patience and flexibility will be vital in adapting to the shifts ahead.

For those born in the year of the Wood Snake (1965), 2025 is a 'Duplicating Zodiac Year,' a concept in Chinese astrology. This means that the energy of the Snake, which is already present in their birth year, will be amplified in 2025. As a result, indecision and restlessness may surface more prominently. Caution is advised, especially in personal well-being and financial matters. Taking risks or breaking the rules may lead to unnecessary complications, so staying grounded and mindful of safety is essential.

While 2025 brings vibrant energy, it also carries hidden tensions and dangers. This year, like the Snake, which is peaceful and harmless unless provoked, reminds us to approach challenges calmly and calmly. Being reactive or impulsive could lead to unnecessary difficulties, so measured responses are crucial.

In contrast to the unpredictable energy of the 2024 Wood Dragon year, which brought dramatic fluctuations and instability, the Wood Snake promises a more grounded and positive energy. While the Wood element continues to influence growth and progress, Fire, a vital energy source for the economy and success, remains less prominent in 2025. The caution for this year is to avoid letting the pursuit of power or success overshadow the quality of life. Striking a balance between ambition and harmony will lead to long-term success.

Like the Wood Dragon of 2024, which fuelled artistic and creative ventures, the Wood Snake in 2025 will encourage quiet innovation, introspection, and inner wisdom. It is a year for personal and spiritual development, where transformation happens beneath the surface. For those aligned with the Snake's energy, the rewards will come through patience, reflection, and a deep connection with one's inner self.

Love and relationships are more reflective and thoughtful in the Year of the Wood Snake. The Snake's quiet wisdom encourages us to nurture connections with patience and care, allowing time for growth and understanding. For those seeking love, 2025 is a year to focus on self-reflection and emotional readiness before embarking on new relationships. Like the delicate vines of Yin Wood, love this year will require nourishment and attention to blossom fully. Relationships built on trust, communication, and shared growth will thrive.

The Wood Snake brings a year of strategic advancement in careers and professional pursuits. This is a time for calculated moves rather than bold, impulsive actions. Those who take the time to assess their long-term goals and make thoughtful decisions will find success. Creativity and innovation will flourish, especially in fields that value intellect and wisdom. While progress may seem slow, the Snake's energy rewards persistence and careful planning. Avoid taking unnecessary risks or making hasty decisions, particularly in financial matters. Collaboration with like-minded individuals will yield the most fruitful results, as teamwork rooted in mutual respect and shared vision will be crucial to career growth in 2025.

On a global scale, 2025 will be marked by a shift towards introspection and subtle but impactful transformations. The Wood Snake's influence will encourage nations and leaders to approach political and social issues cautiously. Diplomatic efforts and peaceful negotiations will be more effective than aggressive approaches. However, hidden tensions may arise, requiring careful handling to avoid more significant conflicts. Societies may see a rise in movements focusing on personal growth, environmental sustainability, and the re-evaluation of traditional power structures. Technological innovation will continue, particularly in areas that promote long-term sustainability and wisdom-based solutions to global challenges. The year offers an opportunity for quiet but meaningful progress on the world stage as long as leaders and citizens approach change with patience and clarity.

The Year of the Wood Snake will be a subtle transformation and growth. Unlike the dynamic and dramatic shifts in the Year of the Wood Dragon, 2025 calls for a more measured approach to life's challenges. Personal development, introspection, and careful planning will lead to success, while impulsive actions may backfire. It is a year for quiet innovation, where progress happens beneath the surface. Patience and thoughtful decision-making will benefit relationships, careers, and global events. While the year may present hidden challenges, those who embrace the wisdom and transformative energy of the Snake will find themselves well-positioned for long-term success and renewal.

CHINESE NEW YEAR TRADITIONS

Key Practices:

Thoroughly clean your home, removing all clutter.

Keep away old brooms and brushes, replacing them with new ones to avert bad luck.

Settle existing debts if possible.

Reconcile any conflicts with family, friends, neighbours, and business partners.

Preparations, Customs, and Superstitions:

Use fresh red envelopes (ang pows) and new banknotes. Stock up on Mandarin oranges.

Display a circular candy tray.

Decorate with flowers like plum blossom, peach blossom, and pussy willow,

symbolising happiness and good fortune. Wear new clothes and shoes for the occasion.

Lunar Chinese New Year Etiquette:

Greet others with "Gong Xi Fa Cai" to wish them a prosperous New Year.

Prepare food in advance to avoid using sharp tools on New Year's Day to preserve luck.

Maintain a positive, joyful atmosphere, refraining from negative expressions.

Avoid washing your hair on the first day of the New Year, as it's associated with

washing away prosperity.

Stick to bright, auspicious colours like red and gold while avoiding white and black.

Exchange Mandarin oranges when visiting, and unmarried individuals receive Hong Baos (Ang POWS) for good luck.

Embracing Lunar Chinese New Year's Significance

Chinese New Year, Lunar Day 1, 2025, falling on January 28th, is a pivotal moment in Chinese culture. The belief is that initiating the year with precise actions, timing, and direction can invite good fortune and prosperity for the year ahead. The tradition involves selecting a specific direction to welcome auspicious stars through prayer offerings from 12:00 a.m. to 12:59 a.m. These stars are aligned with distinct purposes: Wealth resides in the North, the Southeast is for Happiness, the Northeast symbolises Nobility and Patronage, and the East is the doorway to Good Luck. This practice reflects Chinese customs' rich tapestry and deep-rooted connection to auspicious beginnings.

UNVEILING THE CLASH IN 2025

Chinese astrology identifies four Zodiac signs that clash with the Annual Ruling Sign each year. In 2025, these clashing signs are the Tiger, Monkey, Snake, and Pig, collectively known as "Treasure Boxes" in this realm. The severity of these clashes varies depending on an individual's Ba Zi chart. The impact can be more pronounced if two or more Clashing signs are present. The Pig sign faces the most significant challenge due to a direct clash with the Snake sign, potentially introducing changes or obstacles. Individuals with these signs should maintain a low profile, exercise caution, and avoid impulsive decisions to mitigate potential negative consequences, including accidents, conflicts, scandals, health issues, divorce, or financial setbacks.

DECODING THE SIGNIFICANCE OF THE 2025 CLASHES

In 2025, different Chinese Zodiac signs face various types of clashes, each with its recommended resolutions:

For the Tiger, it's a conflict clash; the key is maintaining humility and avoiding conflicts of interest.

The Monkey experiences a direct clash and should opt for a low-profile approach,

steering clear of adventure, rulebreaking, and prioritising personal safety.

If you're a Snake, you encounter an offending clash, making it vital to stay low-key and avoid confrontations and rule-breaking while focusing on personal well-being.

Those born under the Pig sign deal with a penalty clash, which requires self-

discipline, flexibility, and vigilance against betrayal issues.

DISCOVERING THE MOST COMPATIBLE SIGN IN 2025

Each year, one of the 12 zodiac signs aligns harmoniously with the ruling zodiac sign, often referred to as "The Grand Duke" or Tai Shui. In 2025, the Monkey sign claims this favourable position. Per ancient beliefs, carrying a Monkey emblem or symbol can help ward off potential metaphysical ill effects and foster greater harmony and positive energy in your everyday life.

Secret Friends for Your Aid

Secret Friends, zodiac signs that provide support and compatibility, can help counter the metaphysical challenges stemming from clashes with the Grand Duke. They are also believed to attract helpful and supportive individuals into your life. The Secret Friend pairings for the Chinese Lunar Zodiac signs are as follows:

Rat: Ox, Dragon, Monkey   **Ox:** Rat, Snake, Rooster   **Tiger:** Pig, Dog, Horse

Rabbit: Dog, Pig, Goat   **Dragon:** Rooster, Monkey, Rat   **Snake:** Monkey, Rooster, Ox

Horse: Goat, Tiger, Dog   **Goat:** Horse, Rabbit, Pig   **Monkey:** Rat, Dragon, Snake

Rooster: Snake, Ox, Dragon   **Dog:** Rabbit, Horse, Tiger   **Pig:** Tiger, Goat, Rabbit

AUSPICIOUS FENG SHUI COLOURS FOR 2025

Discover the auspicious Feng Shui colours for 2025, the Year of the Wood Snake in Chinese astrology. This year's primary lucky colours, spring green and imperial yellow, are influenced by the elemental themes of Wood and Earth, enhancing luck when used in clothing, accessories, or energy stones. Feng Shui principles consider the annual Flying Stars' positions and room-specific dynamics, guiding interior decor and furniture placement to align with desired energies.

In 2025, each colour will carry specific meanings associated with favoured activities and potential risks.

Blue represents peace and freedom, which makes it ideal for negotiations and job interviews. However, as it's associated with the water element, be cautious of its potential to evoke coldness and laziness.

Green symbolises creativity, healing, and expansion, making it ideal for embarking on new journeys like starting a new job or moving. However, as it's associated with the wood element, be wary of its potential to lead to madness or envy.

Red signifies vital momentum, passion, and love, making it suitable for romantic encounters and celebrating the anticipation of a new baby. However, it's crucial to be alert to its potential for danger and anger, as it's linked to the Fire element. This awareness can help you manage potential conflicts and maintain a balanced emotional state.

Yellow embodies clairvoyance, organisation, and learning, favouring real estate transactions and asset transfers. However, as it's tied to the Earth element, be cautious of its potential for deceit and vanity.

White represents precision, resistance, and equity, making it suitable for commerce, banking, and territorial defence activities. However, it's important to be vigilant and cautious, as it's associated with the metal element and its potential for sorrow and defamation. This understanding can help you navigate potential challenges and maintain your integrity.

To maximise the efficacy of Lucky Colours of 2025, it's recommended that they be considered in mobile contexts, such as personal accessories, vehicles, luggage, or bags, rather than static settings like homes or workplaces.

In 2025, harness the ideal annual colours for each of the 12 Chinese zodiac signs to balance the unique Snake and Wood Yang energy blend. These colours provide protection, boost energy, and attract good fortune, mitigating potential challenges and enhancing determination and success.

Rat:	Fire Red, Burnt Sienna
Ox:	Coral Red, Prussian Blue
Tiger:	Bright Red, Bright Silver
Rabbit	Steel Gray, Scarlet Red
Dragon:	Golden Ochre, Fern Green
Snake:	Midnight Blue, Garnet Red
Horse:	Cinnamon Brown, Vermilion Red
Goat:	Brick Red, Deep Blue
Monkey:	Navy Blue, Earth Brown
Rooster:	Icy White, Yellow Ochre
Dog:	Sapphire Blue, Emerald Green
Pig:	Dark Green, Royal Blue

Fashion Trends in 2025: Under the influence of the Yin Wood Snake, 2025 brings a period of wisdom, introspection, and transformation, reflected in fashion, decor, and celebrations. The 'Wood Snake's energy' refers to the characteristics and influences associated with the Wood Snake in Chinese astrology. This energy favours a thoughtful, strategic approach, emphasising subtlety and elegance in all areas of life. The lucky colours for the year—emerald, green and carmine, red—dominate these spheres, symbolising growth, vitality, passion, and inner change.

As a symbol of metamorphosis, the Wood Snake inspires refined creativity and profound yet discreet transformation. Emerald, green, representing the wood element, embodies renewal, growth, and vitality, while carmine, red, tied to the Snake's intrinsic fire element, signifies passion, energy, and profound personal transformation.

Fashion in 2025 embraces this transformative spirit, with ready-to-wear brands and designers leaning toward more ethical and sustainable practices. The industry is moving toward eco-consciousness, with materials like bamboo, cactus fibres, and organic cotton taking centre stage. Artisanal manufacturing techniques that respect the environment and eco-friendly dyeing and printing processes are increasingly valued to minimise environmental impact.

The Wood element amplifies the desire for pragmatic and creative shifts, driven by the need for meaningful yet quiet change. Under the guidance of the Wood Snake, bold ideas come to fruition, sparking innovation and renewed optimism. This year encourages us to rethink our approach to life with a fresh perspective, incorporating the wisdom and prudence of the Snake. Fusing cultures and ideas will foster deep, constructive dialogues, offering a clear and long-term vision in a rapidly evolving world.

How to use the Complete Feng Shui Planner

Clarity and good timing are vital in ensuring that whatever you undertake is given the best possible chance of success. Even simple everyday activities can have substantial adverse outcomes if riddled with obstacles and bad energy.

ACTIVITY ICONS ❤️ 🏠 ✂️ 🎬 ✈️ 🐕 🚗 🎉 🪨 👙 travelling, moving, renovating, or signing a contract

This planner contains specially calculated auspicious dates for significant activities like cutting your hair, celebrations, travelling, moving, renovating or breaking ground, or signing a contract. Icons on each page mark these.

Understanding The Icons

FAVOURABLE DAYS FOR SPECIFIC TASKS

The icons on each page reveal favourable days for travelling, love and relationship luck, moving house, signing contracts, cutting your hair, buying a car, celebrating, meeting people, starting construction and renovating.

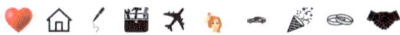

❤️ 🏠 ✂️ 🎬 ✈️ 🐕 🚗 🎉 🪨 👙

Unfavourable days are also indicated for any significant activities on clash days.

⚡

CHINESE ASTROLOGY ANIMALS

Each day's summary includes good /bad days for certain animal signs. When undertaking any significant activity, always check whether it is a good/bad day for your sign, as this overrides whatever the icons indicate. If it is a bad day for the Snake, then all activities will NOT be promising for the Snake that day, no matter what the icons indicate. The Snake must avoid scheduling important issues that day.

FLYING STAR FENG SHUI

Getting your Feng Shui right for the coming year and energising the promising sectors in 2025 will help ensure smooth sailing and a prosperous year ahead.

As we move from one year to the next, energy changes. Transforming from Yin to Yang, from element to element, from one animal sign to the next. Depending on the ruling element and animal, the energy in the home and its occupants also changes from one month to the next. Time exerts a powerful impact on your Feng Shui, luck, and destiny.

Good Feng Shui cannot and does not last forever. It must be recharged with small but significant changes every year. Energy must be refreshed, reorganised and re-energised. Spaces and places need rejuvenation. Energy must be kept moving.

The Flying Stars formula of Feng Shui is a technical approach that directly addresses the effect of time on the energy of homes and businesses and holds a beautiful promise that enables you to improve your luck tremendously. The 2025 Feng Shui chart maps out the distribution of energy in each of the eight sectors of the compass, as well as the centre.

The best strategy is to take care of the negative Stars first and then concentrate on boosting the good ones. Pay closer attention to the sectors where your main door, living room and bedrooms are located. The luck in the main entrance and living room sector affects everyone in the household, while the bedroom alters the fate of those who sleep in it.

The Flying Star energy undergoes annual changes, and a dominant star positioned at the centre of the Lo Shu chart governs the overall energy for the year. In 2025, the reigning Flying Star is the 2, while different stars influence specific sectors. For instance, the WW is impacted by the Flying Star 3, the NE by the Flying Star 4, and so on. Additionally, the Flying Stars' energy varies monthly as a new star joins the annual stars, influencing each month's energy. You can find a monthly overview at the start of each month. Furthermore, a daily Flying Star number reflects the energy of the day. Understanding the meaning and energy of the Flying Stars allows you to assess the daily quality of luck.

FAVOURABLE STARS

1 Victory Triumph and Success Star (Water Element): Helps attain victory over competition and enhances career promotion and monetary growth. Strengthen and improve energy by placing a Victory Horse, Ruyi, or Dragon Tortoise. A water feature would also be incredibly beneficial.

2 Rebirth and Positive Change (Earth Element): This Star supports health growth and well-being, bringing improvement to physical ailments and diseases. . . Support the energy by placing a Wu Lou (Health Gourd), Six Gold Coins on a red tassel, a Saltwater Cure and a Quan Yin in the Southwest.

4 Romance and Literacy Star (Wood Element): Good Star improves relationship opportunities, study, and literary fortune for writers and scholars. Enhance luck with bright lights, fire energy, and wood energy: Place Mandarin Ducks or Huggers, peach blossom animals, plants and fresh flowers in this area.

6 Heavenly Luck Star (Metal Element): Associated with good fortune and help from heaven, it brings speculative luck, power, and authority. Use bright lights, a water feature and Metal to enhance, such as Six Gold Coins on red tassels and Gold Ingots within this area. A Horse will also assist.

8 Retired Prosperity Star (Earth Element): Signifies steady wealth, prosperity, success and happiness. Strengthen and enhance by placing any form of wealth symbolism such as a Buddha, Wealth God, Six Gold Coins on a red tassel, and Gold Ingots.

9 Multiplying Current Prosperity Star (Fire Element): Signifies future prosperity; spurs celebrations, festivities, gatherings and excellent good luck. Enhance with red accessories, bright lights, or any wealth symbolism such as a Buddha, a Wealth God, 9 Gold Coins on a red tassel, or Gold Ingots.

UNFAVOURABLE STARS

3 Hostile, Conflict and Dispute Star (Wood Element): An evil Star signifies lawsuits, hostility and quarrels. Brings misunderstandings among staff, clients and colleagues and trouble with the authorities. I recommend placing Fire energy in this area, such as bright lights or a red piece of paper, or you can use any red décor object. If your front door is in this area, I recommend placing Temple Lions and the Evil Eye symbol. Remove any excess water or plants. Remove Metal windchimes. Do not overstimulate with radio or TV energy.

5 Misfortune and Obstacles Star (Earth Element), also known as Wu Wang or 5 Yellow Star: It is considered the most vicious and dangerous of the nine Stars; it brings all kinds of misfortunes, accidents, losses and death. Subdue with a Brass 5-element Pagoda and a Saltwater Cure in the centre. A Ganesha will also assist with the removal of obstacles. Keep electrical equipment to a minimum and avoid the colours red and yellow. Try to avoid any significant activity within this sector.

7 Robbery and Evil Star (Metal Element): This unlucky star brings loss, robbery, violence, and gossip to the West sector. Suppress by placing three pieces of Lucky Bamboo in a vase of water and bright lights in this area, along with the Evil Eye

Symbol, one Blue Rhinoceros and one Blue Elephant, or two Blue Rhinoceroses for extra protection. If your front door is located here, I also recommend Temple Lions.

2025 AFFLICTIONS

In 2025, the Southeast (105 - 135) will be the designated location of the Tai Sui, also known as the Grand Duke, for the year. The Grand Duke is considered a celestial entity deserving of respect and should not be disturbed or confronted. Significant renovations or earthmoving in this sector are highly recommended to be avoided throughout the year and to maintain a sense of tranquillity in this area. Placing a Chi Lin, Pi Yao, and Fu Dog in the Southeast, facing the Northwest, can help appease and harmonise this sector, but it's best to avoid disturbances altogether.

In 2025, the East will be influenced by the presence of the Three Killings, a challenging energy that can cause health issues and conflicts if disturbed. To minimise its negative impact, it is advised not to sit with your back to the East; instead, face this direction while keeping your back toward the West. Major renovations or earthmoving activities in the East should be avoided to maintain a harmonious atmosphere.

To neutralise the effects of the Three Killings, a common remedy is to place a set of Three Celestial Guardians—such as the Qilin, Fu Dog, and Pi Xiu—in the East sector of your home or workplace. Additionally, lighting up this area with a bright lamp or hanging a metal wind chime can further help to diminish the energy. However, the best approach is to avoid disturbing this sector altogether.

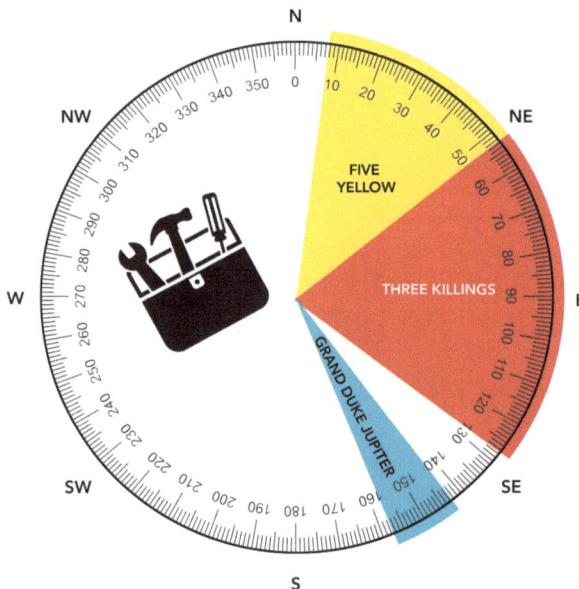

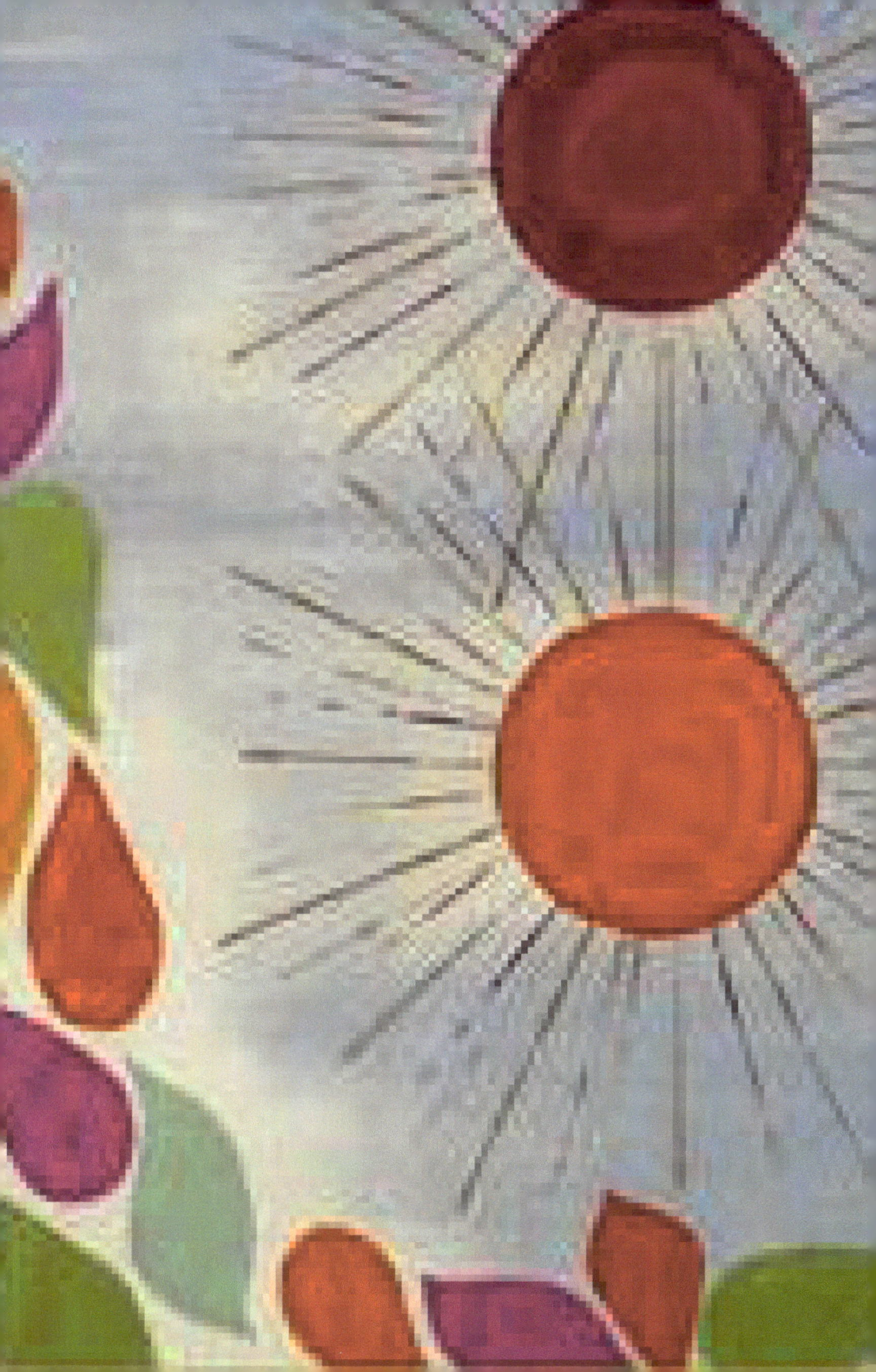

January 6 – February 3 is the Month of the Ox

Ox Chinese Horoscope 2025: Navigating Challenges and Opportunities

Ox Birth Years: 1925, 1937, 1949, 1961, 1973, 1985, 1997, 2009, 2021, 2033

In 2025, the dynamic and transformative energy of the Yin Wood Fire Snake will significantly influence the Ox. As an embodiment of steadfastness and perseverance, the Ox will find itself in a year filled with change and opportunities. The Fire Snake's intense energy urges Oxen to adapt, evolve, and embrace new possibilities.

Fire Snake Influence: Passion and Transformation

The Fire Snake's influence in 2025 brings a transformative energy that pushes Oxen to step out of their comfort zones. This year will require adaptability, with the Fire Snake encouraging Oxen to embrace passion, creativity, and innovation. While challenges may arise, the Snake's energy will drive Oxen to navigate these obstacles with resilience and strategic thinking.

Career Prospects 2025: Embracing Change and Growth

In 2025, the Fire Snake's influence will propel Oxen toward new career opportunities and professional growth. This is a year to explore new ventures and be open to change. The Snake's energy will support Oxen in showcasing their skills and adaptability. Fields such as technology, media, and the arts may offer significant opportunities for advancement. Collaboration and building strong professional relationships will be crucial to success.

Financial Outlook: Strategic Planning and Stability

Financially, the Year of the Fire Snake emphasises the importance of strategic planning and cautious decision-making. While opportunities for financial growth will arise, Oxen should avoid impulsive investments and focus on long-term strategies. The Snake's energy favours careful budgeting and prudent spending. Seeking expert advice and avoiding unnecessary risks will ensure financial stability.

Love and Relationships: Passion and Depth

In Love, 2025, brings passion and intensity to the Ox. Existing relationships may deepen, with the Fire Snake's influence encouraging emotional growth and connection. The year offers new romantic possibilities for single Oxen, but choosing partners wisely and prioritising emotional compatibility is essential. The Fire Snake's energy will enhance the Ox's natural loyalty and reliability, leading to meaningful and lasting relationships.

Health and Wellness: Maintaining Balance

The intense energy of the Fire Snake calls for a balanced approach to health and well-being. Oxen should prioritise self-care by incorporating regular exercise, a balanced diet, and stress management into their routines. The Snake's influence may bring emotional highs and lows, so focusing on mental and emotional health is essential. Activities such as meditation and mindfulness practices can help maintain equilibrium.

Symbolism of the Ox and Fire Snake: Transformation and Renewal

The Ox's grounded nature meets the Fire Snake's transformative and passionate energy in 2025. This combination symbolises a year of renewal and growth. By embracing the Fire Snake's vibrant energy, Oxen can achieve personal and professional transformation.

2025: A Year of Passion and Growth

The Year of the Yin Wood Fire Snake offers Oxen a dynamic and transformative journey. Embrace the opportunities for change and growth by adapting to new situations, pursuing innovative ideas, and maintaining a balanced approach to finances and health. With careful planning and an open mind, Oxen can turn challenges into opportunities for success and advancement in 2025.

JANUARY Flying Star 3, Discord, Conflict, and Caution

January begins the year under a cloud of discord as Flying Star 3 makes its ominous entrance into the celestial ballet. This star brings a surge of turbulent energies, vibrating with the unsettling resonance of conflict and strife. However, it's important to remember that there is potential for positive change even amid this turbulence. In its wake, seeds of gossip, disputes, and legal challenges find fertile ground, sprouting into full-blown turmoil. Far from benign, Flying Star 3 is a force of hostility, notorious for weaving a complex tapestry of violence, anger, and endless disagreements. It heralds a storm of misunderstandings, igniting fiery arguments and even litigation, casting a dark shadow over relationships between family members, friends, and colleagues.

The health ramifications that accompany this star are equally foreboding. It targets the liver, gallbladder, feet, and arms, manifesting in physical discomfort and malaise. As its influence spreads, productivity may falter, with the atmosphere thickening under the weight of conflict and friction.

Particularly vulnerable are those born in the Year of the Dog and Pig and the male head of the household. Marital bonds and familial harmony become entangled in the web of Flying Star 3's disruptive energies. The tension it fosters can cast a long shadow over relationships between spouses, eroding the foundations of stability within families and marriages. The looming threat of conflict with authorities and potential legal entanglements is a stark reminder of the need for heightened caution during this period. It's crucial to be alert and prepared, as this caution can help us navigate the challenges of Flying Star 3 with resilience and strength.

Under the influence of Flying Star 3, January demands a vigilant and defensive approach. However, it's important to remember that various remedies can counteract its negative energy. The traditional Chinese cure—a simple red piece of paper—can be a powerful tool to ward off its malign influence. Surroundings can be imbued with the protective energies of red and purple, introduced through decor, candles, and bright lights. The magic flaming wheel, a symbolic shield, can also be invoked to fend off negativity. Images of the fiery red phoenix or the watchful eagle can be guardians, defending against discord. For those seeking an extra layer of protection, the steadfast presence of temple lions and the vigilant gaze of the evil eye symbol can be enlisted, ensuring that the darkness remains at bay. These remedies offer a beacon of hope, empowering us to navigate the challenges of Flying Star 3 with resilience and strength.

In 2025, the Northwest sector will be particularly significant for feng shui enhancements. According to the Luo Shu or Bagua School of Feng Shui, this area is governed by the annual Flying Star 3, which symbolises critical figures such as the man of the house, influential benefactors, mentors, and supportive individuals. Focusing on this sector can strengthen personal and professional relationships, encouraging and motivating homeowners.

The Northwest is associated with the Metal element, which, in Chinese culture, signifies gold and family wealth. To harness and amplify this energy, incorporate metal décor items, objects in metallic colours, bells, or wind chimes. Additionally, placing the three Star Gods—representing health, wealth, and longevity—in the main living area can substantially benefit all household members, fostering a harmonious and prosperous environment.

The Wood Snake Year

30 Monday

Animal: **Earth Dragon**
Flying Star: **5**
Good Day: **Rooster**
Bad Day: **Dog**

31 Tuesday

Animal: **Earth Snake**
Flying Star: **6**
Good Day: **Monkey**
Bad Day: **Pig**

1 Wednesday

Animal: **Metal Horse**
Flying Star: **7**
Good Day: **Goat**
Bad Day: **Rat**

2 Thursday

Animal: **Metal Goat**
Flying Star: **8**
Good Day: **Horse**
Bad Day: **Ox**
✈ 🐴🏫

3 Friday

Animal: **Water Monkey**
Flying Star: **9**
Good Day: **Snake**
Bad Day: **Tiger**
✈ 🏠🪙

4 Saturday

Animal: **Water Rooster**
Flying Star: **1**
Good Day: **Dragon**
Bad Day: **Rabbit**
🐴

5 Sunday

Animal: **Wood Dog**
Flying Star: **2**
Good Day: **Rabbit**
Bad Day: **Dragon**
🪙

JANUARY MONTHLY CHINESE ZODIAC OVERVIEW

RAT

After a fulfilling and dynamic year, it's time to reflect and set new goals for 2025. Focus on maintaining strong ethics in your business endeavours, which will enhance decision-making. As the new Lunar Year unfolds, prioritise rest and wellness to recharge your energy reserves.

OX

2024 brought a mix of highs and challenges. With lessons learned, you're well-equipped to enter the new Lunar Year. The month will be busy with work, but take advantage of the vibrant energy and ensure you recharge yourself.

TIGER

There's still unfinished work as the Dragon year wraps up. This month brings harmonious energy, making it an ideal time to focus on well-being. Ensure you're revitalised and ready for the opportunities of the new Lunar Year.

RABBIT

January's energy will uplift both your physical and emotional well-being. As activities ramp up, focus on self-care to stay energised and prepared for the new Lunar Year.

DRAGON

Though the Dragon year had twists, you've navigated through with strength. It's time to set fresh intentions for the new Lunar Year. Positive changes are ahead, and well-being remains a key priority.

SNAKE

2024 may have been tiring, but it brought rewards. As you step into the new Lunar Year, anxieties will ease. Focus on self-care, pampering, and enjoying social activities. In business, avoid impulsive decisions and stick to tried strategies for success.

HORSE

Reflect on your journey as you transition into the new Lunar Year. New possibilities are on the horizon, so take time to set clear goals and financial plans. Recharge your energy for the busy year ahead.

The Wood Snake Year

6
Monday

Animal: **Wood Pig**
Flying Star: **3**
Good Day: **Tiger**
Bad Day: **Snake**
✈ ︎🎉

7
Tuesday

Animal: **Fire Rat**
Flying Star: **4**
Good Day: **Ox**
Bad Day: **Horse**

8
Wednesday

Animal: **Fire Ox**
Flying Star: **5**
Good Day: **Rat**
Bad Day: **Goat**

9
Thursday

Animal: **Earth Tiger**
Flying Star: **6**
Good Day: **Pig**
Bad Day: **Monkey**

10
Friday

Animal: **Earth Rabbit**
Flying Star: **7**
Good Day: **Dog**
Bad Day: **Rooster**

11
Saturday

Animal: **Metal Dragon**
Flying Star: **8**
Good Day: **Rooster**
Bad Day: **Dog**

12
Sunday

Animal: **Metal Snake**
Flying Star: **9**
Good Day: **Monkey**
Bad Day: **Pig**

GOAT

As the Lunar Year changes, dedicate this month to yourself. Self-care activities like yoga, meditation, or time in nature will be particularly beneficial, helping you relax and rejuvenate.

MONKEY

Prepare for further transformations as you step into the new Lunar Year. Travel and new work opportunities may arise, so stay open to adjustments and embrace the changes flexibly.

ROOSTER

The Dragon Year has brought growth and personal development. Now is the time to review your plans and prepare for the following year. Reflect on the paths that will lead to further success.

DOG

2024 may have been uncomfortable, but it has fuelled your growth. As the new Lunar Year begins, harmony and rewards await you. Embrace the optimism and confidence of the year ahead.

PIG

Dynamic energy flows smoothly into the new Lunar Year. While you've enjoyed your achievements, 2025 is a clashing year for your sign. Pace yourself, focusing on wellness and balance for continued success.

01 | JANUARY 2025

The Wood Snake Year

13
Monday

Animal: **Water Horse**
Flying Star: **1**
Good Day: **Goat**
Bad Day: **Rat**

14
Tuesday

Animal: **Water Goat**
Flying Star: **2**
Good Day: **Horse**
Bad Day: **Ox**

15
Wednesday

Animal: **Wood Monkey**
Flying Star: **3**
Good Day: **Snake**
Bad Day: **Tiger**

16
Thursday

Animal: **Wood Rooster**
Flying Star: **4**
Good Day: **Dragon**
Bad Day: **Rabbit**

17
Friday

Animal: **Fire Dog**
Flying Star: **5**
Good Day: **Rabbit**
Bad Day: **Dragon**

18
Saturday

Animal: **Fire Pig**
Flying Star: **6**
Good Day: **Tiger**
Bad Day: **Snake**

19
Sunday

Animal: **Earth Rat**
Flying Star: **7**
Good Day: **Ox**
Bad Day: **Horse**

THE FENG SHUI OF YOUR FRONT DOOR

The significance of the main entrance cannot be overstated, as it serves as the gateway for chi, the vital life force energy, to enter your home. The condition of the chi surrounding your front door can influence the energy within, impacting the well-being of all occupants. Assessing and enhancing the feng shui of your main door is a pivotal step in fostering positive energy flow.

Eliminate any potential 'poison arrows' directed at your main door. Be vigilant for sharp edges and triangular rooflines pointing towards the entrance. If feasible, consider relocating the main door to a more favourable position to avoid negative energy influences.

Avoid positioning the main door beneath a bathroom. If this configuration exists, consider moving the entrance to a different area along the frontage to mitigate any adverse effects.

Ensure that the main door does not directly face narrow gaps between buildings. Such an alignment may lead to health issues and financial setbacks. Opt for a relocation if necessary.

Keep the area around the main door clean and unobstructed. Avoid placing shoes directly before the entrance to maintain a smooth, positive energy flow.

Allow some open space in front of the main door to facilitate the pooling and gentle energy flow into your home. This practice is believed to attract good luck and positive vibes.

Ensure the main door is proportionate to the size of your house. A considerable door may contribute to financial challenges, while a door that is too small can disrupt familial harmony. Strive for a balanced and harmonious entrance that complements the overall scale of your home.

01 | JANUARY 2025

The Wood Snake Year

20
Monday

Animal: **Earth Ox**
Flying Star: **8**
Good Day: **Rat**
Bad Day: **Goat**

21
Tuesday

Animal: **Metal Tiger**
Flying Star: **9**
Good Day: **Pig**
Bad Day: **Monkey**

22
Wednesday

Animal: **Metal Rabbit**
Flying Star: **1**
Good Day: **Dog**
Bad Day: **Rooster**

23
Thursday

Animal: **Water Dragon**
Flying Star: **2**
Good Day: **Rooster**
Bad Day: **Dog**

24
Friday

Animal: **Water Snake**
Flying Star: **3**
Good Day: **Monkey**
Bad Day: **Pig**

25
Saturday

Animal: **Wood Pig**
Flying Star: **4**
Good Day: **Tiger**
Bad Day: **Snake**

26
Sunday

Animal: **Wood Rat**
Flying Star: **5**
Good Day: **Ox**
Bad Day:z **Horse**

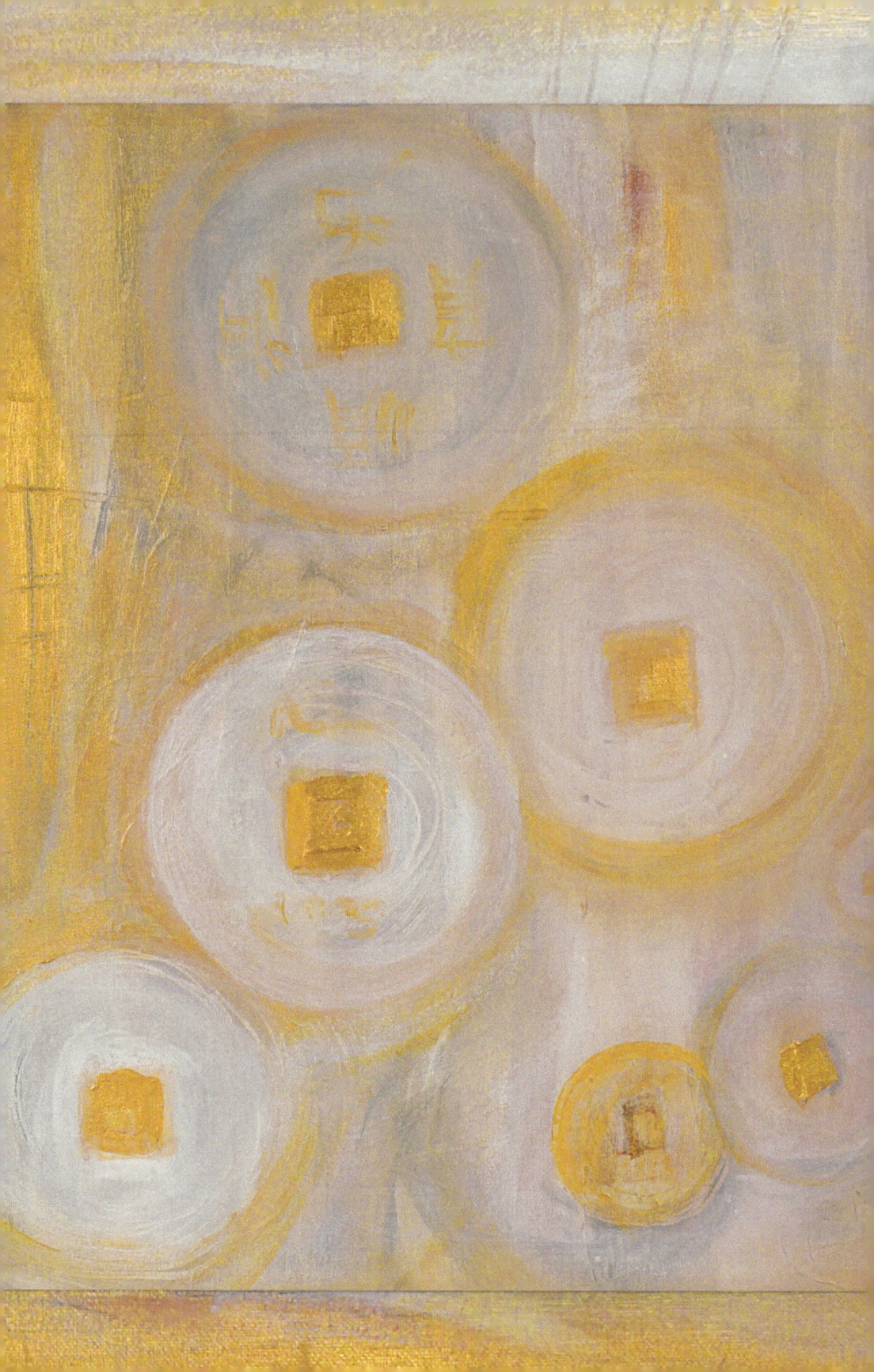

01 | JANUARY 2025

The Wood Snake Year

27
Monday

Animal: **Fire Ox**
Flying Star: **6**
Good Day: **Rat**
Bad Day: **Goat**

28
Tuesday

Animal: **Fire Tiger**
Flying Star: **7**
Good Day: **Pig**
Bad Day: **Monkey**

29
Wednesday

Animal: **Earth Rabbit**
Flying Star: **8**
Good Day: **Dog**
Bad Day: **Rooster**

30
Thursday

Animal: **Earth Dragon**
Flying Star: **9**
Good Day: **Rooster**
Bad Day: **Dog**

31
Friday

Animal: **Metal Snake**
Flying Star: **1**
Good Day: **Monkey**
Bad Day: **Pig**

1
Saturday

Animal: **Metal Ox**
Flying Star: **2**
Good Day: **Rat**
Bad Day: **Goat**

2
Sunday

Animal: **Water Tiger**
Flying Star: **3**
Good Day: **Pig**
Bad Day: **Monkey**

February 4 - March 5 is the Month of the Tiger

Tiger Chinese Horoscope 2025: Navigating Challenges and Prosperity

Tiger Birth Years: 1926, 1938, 1950, 1962, 1974, 1986, 1998, 2010, 2022, 2034

In 2025, the Tiger encounters the transformative energies of the Yin Wood-Snake. This contrasts with the previous Yang Wood Earth Dragon, shifting the dynamics and introducing new challenges and opportunities. The Fire Snake's influence calls for adaptability and careful navigation throughout the year.

Financial Outlook: Caution and Vigilance

Due to the Fire Snake's intense energy, the Tiger's financial landscape 2025 is marked by potential volatility. Avoid risky investments and be meticulous with budgeting. Business ventures should be approached with caution, prioritising safety and due diligence. Unexpected financial fluctuations may arise, so maintaining a conservative financial strategy is essential.

Career Progress and Artistic Fields

For Tigers involved in creative and artistic pursuits, 2025 offers promising prospects. The Fire Snake's influence can ignite inspiration and lead to success in artistic endeavours. Skilful presentation and leveraging creative talents will open career growth and recognition doors.

Mixed Love Fortunes: Patience and Communication

The year brings a blend of experiences in matters of love. Single Tigers may encounter potential partners, but a cautious, measured approach is advised. Those in relationships might experience communication challenges; addressing these through open dialogue and patience will strengthen bonds. Married Tigers should focus on shared activities to enhance relationship stability.

Positive Career Prospects: Empowerment and Humility

Despite potential career hurdles, the year holds positive prospects. Tigers' diligence and dedication will lead to new opportunities and recognition. Balancing assertiveness with humility will ensure a well-rounded career advancement approach, fostering respect and success.

Favourable Finance Opportunities: Planning and Restraint

Financial stability for Tigers in 2025 hinges on disciplined planning and restraint. Avoid impulsive spending and focus on strategic investments. A conservative approach will safeguard against unexpected expenses and promote steady economic growth.

Holistic Health: Routine and Well-being

Maintaining a disciplined routine, including regular exercise and mindfulness practices, is crucial for Tigers' well-being. The intense energy of the Fire Snake necessitates careful stress management. Practices such as meditation, yoga, or Tai Chi will support physical and mental health. Avoiding harmful habits and nurturing resilience will be beneficial.

Snake and Tiger Harmony: Mutual Benefit

The Tiger's Yin Wood energy interacts uniquely with the Fire Snake's elements. This relationship encourages personal growth and transformation. While the Snake's fiery nature introduces challenges, it also offers development opportunities. Embrace this dynamic interplay to enhance both personal and professional aspects of life.

2025: The Power of Tiger and Fire Snake

The Year of the Yin Wood Snake represents a profound change and opportunity for the Tiger. By leveraging adaptability, patience, and strategic planning, Tigers can navigate the year's challenges and capitalise on potential growth. Embrace the Fire Snake's energy for transformation and success.

Snake and Tiger Synergy: Prosperity and Success

The interplay between the Tiger and the Fire Snake's energies highlights a year of significant transformation and opportunity. By collaborating harmoniously and embracing change, Tigers can navigate challenges effectively and achieve success across various aspects of life.

FEBRUARY Flying Star 2: From Turmoil to Complex Energies

February ushers in the complex energies of Flying Star 2, a star that straddles both the remnants of its past and the promise of its future. As the cosmic dance continues, Star 2 takes place on the celestial stage, undergoing a profound metamorphosis that began in February 2024. While it now carries a glimmer of promising potential, the star's energy remains weak and still harbours the power of sickness and illness, a reminder of its turbulent legacy.

This transformation marks a significant shift in the cosmic landscape. Once a harbinger of affliction and negative energy during Period 8, Flying Star 2 is gradually shedding its inauspicious cloak as we progress into Period 9. Like a phoenix rising from the ashes, it embodies a new role as a force for positive change, although its influence remains cautious and tentative. Health and well-being, once threatened by this star, are now on the cusp of improvement, though the shadow of its past still lingers.

In Period 9, Flying Star 2 retains its Earth element, wielding energies that once wreaked havoc on health and peace. The early phases of this transition are marked by residual turbulence as the star's influence continues to present challenges, albeit less severe than in the past.

For 2025, Star 2's presence is felt in every home and building, casting a subtle but undeniable influence on the lives of those it touches. While there may be opportunities in property and real estate endeavours, these gains could come at the expense of health. The toll may be paid through illness or physical discomfort, underscoring the need to carefully manage this star's energy.

To harness Flying Star 2's transformative potential, a range of remedies is recommended. The Health Gourd, or Wu Lou, symbolises healing and well-being, best accompanied by Six Gold Coins on a vibrant red tassel. A Saltwater Cure can help neutralise lingering negative energies, while the presence of Quan Yin invites benevolent vibrations into space. Wearing a Wu Lou pendant or amulet is a protective talisman, particularly for those with low life force energy, shielding them from the star's lingering effects.

Metal elements play a crucial role in counteracting the challenges posed by Flying Star 2. Brass, copper, bronze, and pewter objects, artworks, and decor items introduce stability and balance into the environment. Incorporating white, silver, and gold shades further harmonises the space with the star's evolving energy in Period 9, aligning interiors with its subtle yet significant transformation.

In 2025, the annual Flying Star 2 will influence the Centre sector of the Luo Shu or Bagua School of Feng Shui. This sector is crucial for nurturing health and well-being, encompassing physical, emotional, and spiritual dimensions.

The centre of your home should remain open and unobstructed to ensure a healthy energy flow. Any blockages, such as those caused by staircases or bathrooms, can disrupt this flow. To counteract these issues, the area should be infused with the grounding energy of the Earth Element. Employ square shapes, earthy tones like yellow and tan, and materials such as ceramic tiles to restore balance and enhance vitality.

SE	S	SW
1 **1**	6 **6**	8 **8**
9 **9**	2 **2**	4 **4**
5 **5**	7 **7**	3 **3**

The Wood Snake Year

3
Monday

Animal: **Water Rabbit**
Flying Star: **4**
Good Day: **Dog**
Bad Day: **Rooster**

4
Tuesday

Animal: **Wood Dragon**
Flying Star: **5**
Good Day: **Rooster**
Bad Day: **Dog**

5
Wednesday

Animal: **Wood Snake**
Flying Star: **6**
Good Day: **Monkey**
Bad Day: **Pig**

6
Thursday

Animal: **Fire Horse**
Flying Star: **7**
Good Day: **Goat**
Bad Day: **Rat**

7
Friday

Animal: **Fire Goat**
Flying Star: **8**
Good Day: **Horse**
Bad Day: **Ox**

8
Saturday

Animal: **Earth Monkey**
Flying Star: **9**
Good Day: **Snake**
Bad Day: **Tiger**

9
Sunday

Animal: **Earth Rooster**
Flying Star: **1**
Good Day: **Dragon**
Bad Day: **Rabbit**

FEBRUARY MONTHLY CHINESE ZODIAC OVERVIEW

RAT

This month brings joy and abundance, making it perfect for reconnecting with family and friends. At work, finish pending tasks to prepare for new opportunities. Financial prospects are strong, but be mindful of fatigue and ensure you rest adequately.

OX

This month's energy is unstable, so staying practical is essential. Employers may face staff challenges, and overworking your team could lead to burnout. Take care to maintain balance in your work environment and be considerate of others.

TIGER

You're entering this Lunar Year on a busy note. Both your work and home life will keep you on your toes. Stay open to new ideas and seek advice from experienced colleagues. Financial energy is vital, so expect positive gains.

RABBIT

Optimism returns with the new Lunar Year, but be cautious with your finances. Money energy is weak, so manage spending wisely. Focus on wellness and avoid overindulgence to maintain your balance.

DRAGON

This month's pace slows, allowing you to break bad habits and plan for the future. Financially, now is the time to create solid plans for the years ahead. Use this stability to your advantage.

SNAKE

February brings conflict and discomfort. Be prepared at work, especially with new projects. Avoid hasty career decisions and seek clarity on what you truly want before making any moves.

HORSE

This is a time to slow down and relax after a hectic few months. Avoid workplace conflicts and allow energy to flow naturally. Your energy may dip mid-month, so rest and recharge when needed.

10
Monday

Animal: **Metal Dog**
Flying Star: **2**
Good Day: **Rabbit**
Bad Day: **Dragon**

11
Tuesday

Animal: **Metal Pig**
Flying Star: **3**
Good Day: **Tiger**
Bad Day: **Snake**

12
Wednesday

Animal: **Water Rat**
Flying Star: **4**
Good Day: **Ox**
Bad Day: **Horse**

13
Thursday

Animal: **Water Ox**
Flying Star: **5**
Good Day: **Rat**
Bad Day: **Goat**

14
Friday

Animal: **Wood Tiger**
Flying Star: **6**
Good Day: **Pig**
Bad Day: **Monkey**

15
Saturday

Animal: **Wood Rabbit**
Flying Star: **7**
Good Day: **Dog**
Bad Day: **Rooster**

16
Sunday

Animal: **Fire Dragon**
Flying Star: **8**
Good Day: **Rooster**
Bad Day: **Dog**

GOAT

February starts strong with favourable energy. Identify your goals early to make the most of this month's momentum. Luck is on your side, and relationships will experience harmony, making this a joyous time for both work and love.

MONKEY

February may be demanding, but new opportunities await. Stress in personal relationships could lead to changes, so keep communication calm and avoid unnecessary conflict to maintain harmony.

ROOSTER

The month begins with introspection; being open to new ideas will bring opportunities. Financial energy is favourable, but avoid overextending yourself. Exercise caution in investments and remain grounded in your decision-making.

DOG

February's fluctuating energy may create challenges, but your sensitivity will help you navigate them. Work obstacles will be resolved quickly if approached with focus. Maintain your well-being through consistent exercise and rest.

PIG

This month, supportive energy flows, making it an excellent time for progress. If you are travelling, take extra care with personal safety. Avoid engaging in risky activities and prioritise balance in all areas of life.

17
Monday

Animal: **Fire Snake**
Flying Star: **9**
Good Day: **Monkey**
Bad Day: **Pig**

18
Tuesday

Animal: **Earth Horse**
Flying Star: **1**
Good Day: **Goat**
Bad Day: **Rat**
🏠 🛬 ✈️ 🎉

19
Wednesday

Animal: **Earth Goat**
Flying Star: **2**
Good Day: **Horse**
Bad Day: **Ox**
🪢 🎬

20
Thursday

Animal: **Metal Monkey**
Flying Star: **3**
Good Day: **Snake**
Bad Day: **Tiger**

21
Friday

Animal: **Metal Rooster**
Flying Star: **4**
Good Day: **Dragon**
Bad Day: **Rabbit**
🎬 ❤️ 🖤

22
Saturday

Animal: **Water Dog**
Flying Star: **5**
Good Day: **Rabbit**
Bad Day: **Dragon**
⚡ 🎬

23
Sunday

Animal: **Water Pig**
Flying Star: **6**
Good Day: **Tiger**
Bad Day: **Snake**
🦰

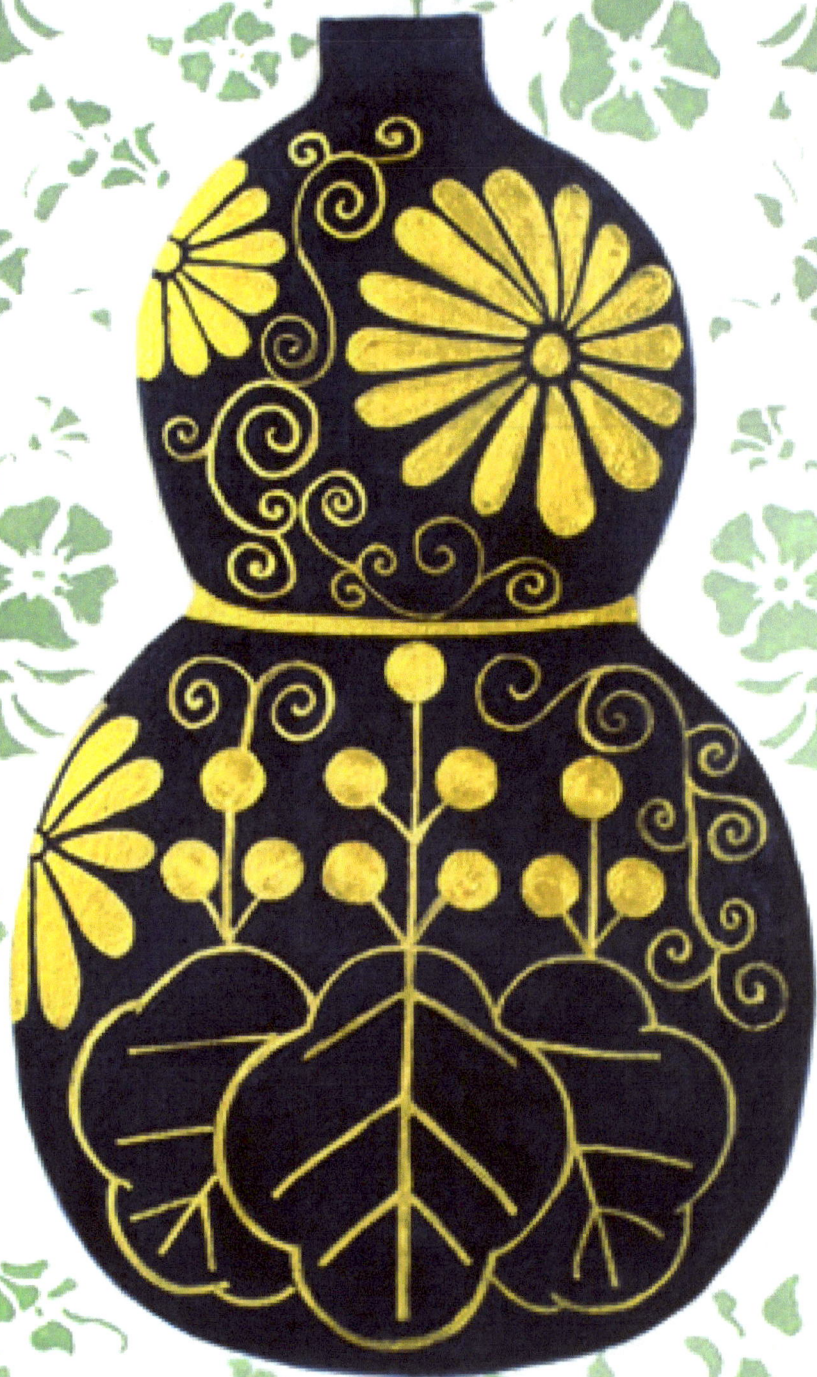

The Wood Snake Year

24
Monday

Animal: **Wood Rat**
Flying Star: **7**
Good Day: **Ox**
Bad Day: **Horse**

25
Tuesday

Animal: **Wood Ox**
Flying Star: **8**
Good Day: **Rat**
Bad Day: **Goat**

26
Wednesday

Animal: **Fire Tiger**
Flying Star: **9**
Good Day: **Pig**
Bad Day: **Monkey**

27
Thursday

Animal: **Fire Rabbit**
Flying Star: **1**
Good Day: **Dog**
Bad Day: **Rooster**

28
Friday

Animal: **Earth Dragon**
Flying Star: **2**
Good Day: **Rooster**
Bad Day: **Dog**

1
Saturday

Animal: **Earth Snake**
Flying Star: **3**
Good Day: **Monkey**
Bad Day: **Pig**

2
Sunday

Animal: **Metal Horse**
Flying Star: **4**
Good Day: **Goat**
Bad Day: **Rat**

March 6 – April 4 is the Month of the Rabbit

Rabbit Chinese Horoscope 2025: Navigating Challenges and Embracing Opportunities

Rabbit Birth Years: **1915, 1927, 1939, 1951, 1963, 1975, 1987, 1999, 2011, 2023, 2035**

In 2025, the Rabbit encounters the dynamic energies of the Yin Wood-Snake. This shifts from the previous year's Earth Dragon influence, bringing new challenges and opportunities. The Fire Snake's transformative and intense nature will significantly impact the Rabbit's year.

Rabbit-Snake Dynamic: Harmony and Transformation

The Fire Snake's presence introduces both harmony and challenge for the Rabbit. While the Rabbit's Wood element aligns with the Snake's Yin Wood, the snake's fiery and passionate nature can create intense dynamics in personal and professional relationships. This alignment fosters growth but may also bring about tension that requires careful management.

Career Outlook: Opportunities and Obstacles

In 2025, career prospects for Rabbits are promising but come with potential hurdles. The Fire Snake's energy can ignite new opportunities and increase competition and demands. Rabbits should focus on skill enhancement and strategic networking. They should avoid unnecessary conflicts and stay adaptable to navigate career challenges effectively.

Love Prospects: Growth and Communication

The year offers a mixed landscape for romance. The Rabbit's natural charm and the Snake's fiery energy create an environment ripe for meaningful connections. Singles may find potential partners, but patience and clear communication are essential. For committed Rabbits, nurturing relationships through open dialogue and shared activities will foster stability and growth.

Financial Gains: Caution and Strategy

Financial prospects are optimistic in 2025, yet the Snake's intense energy calls for caution. Avoid impulsive investments and conduct thorough research before making financial decisions. Strategic planning and disciplined spending will help secure and grow wealth throughout the year.

Wellness and Balance: Mind and Body Integration

Maintaining health and wellness is crucial with the Fire Snake's vibrant influence. Balance emotional and physical well-being through regular exercise, meditation, and a balanced lifestyle. Vigilance against stress and adopting a proactive approach to health will ensure overall vitality.

Rabbit and Snake Partnership: Prosperity and Challenge

The Rabbit's harmonious Wood element interacts with the Snake's dynamic energy, promoting personal and professional growth. This partnership requires balancing the Snake's intense drive with the Rabbit's thoughtful and observant nature. Embrace the transformation and opportunities presented by this synergy.

Holistic Prosperity: Growth and Investment

The Fire Snake year offers substantial financial opportunities. Focus on cautious investments and strategic planning to maximise potential gains. The Rabbit's persistence and adaptability, combined with the Snake's transformative influence, can lead to significant achievements.

Health and Vitality: Mindful Practices

Balance the Rabbit's natural tendencies with the Snake's energetic influence to enhance holistic health. Engage in mindfulness practices, maintain a disciplined routine, and proactively address emotional stress. This balanced approach supports overall well-being and resilience.

Rabbit and Snake Unity: Achievement and Success

The blend of the Rabbit's artistic sensibilities and the Snake's transformative power heralds a year of achievement. Rabbits can achieve success and personal growth by navigating challenges with adaptability and embracing opportunities.

Snake and Rabbit Compatibility: Growth and Harmony

The Fire Snake's influence brings a mix of harmony and intensity to the Rabbit's year. This combination fosters growth and transformation as long as the Rabbit remains adaptable and proactive in managing the dynamic energies.

Chinese Zodiac Rabbit: Embracing Transformation

The Rabbit's journey in the Year of the Yin Wood Snake is marked by significant change and opportunity. While challenges may arise, the Rabbit's ability to adapt and harness the Snake's energy will lead to growth and success.

2025: Rabbit and Snake Synergy

The collaboration between the Rabbit and the Fire Snake sets the stage for a transformative and prosperous year. Embrace the challenges, leverage the opportunities, and navigate the dynamic energy to achieve a successful and fulfilling year.

MARCH Flying Star 1: Triumph, Victory, and Brilliance

March brings forth the luminous energy of Flying Star 1, a beacon of positivity in the cosmic tapestry. Known as the Star of Triumph, this celestial force radiates its benevolent influence across fame, wealth, intelligence, and success. Its presence ushers in a season ripe for growth, achievement, and brilliance, casting a glow of opportunity over all who fall under its light.

With the guiding hand of Flying Star 1, individuals find themselves on pathways to triumph and victory. Its influence reaches far and wide, from elevating careers and reputations to enhancing status and recognition. This star particularly shines in career advancement and academic excellence, fuelling writing, research, and scholarly pursuits. In this celestial symphony, Flying Star 1 creates a harmonious environment where the seeds of success are sown and nurtured to fruition.

The optimism carried by this star is not fleeting; it lays the foundation for enduring triumphs. Whether overcoming competition, realising long-held dreams, or seizing wealth opportunities, the dynamic energy of Flying Star 1 fosters an atmosphere where influence and success flourish. Those aligned with this star, especially the eldest daughter and those born under the Dragon and Snake zodiacs, are encouraged to embrace challenges enthusiastically, knowing victory is within reach.

In addition to its career-enhancing qualities, Flying Star 1 offers a protective shield against health concerns, helping to bolster resilience and vitality. However, it also calls for mindfulness in navigating emotional turbulence. Maintaining emotional stability and guarding against depression is essential during this period, as the star's energy can amplify both positive and negative states.

Flying Star 1's elemental essence is Water, and it channels its triumph through this fluid and powerful conduit. Activating its potential involves introducing Yang energy, symbolised through metallic elements like wind chimes, collections of trophies, or medals that resonate with the star's victorious spirit. Flowing water features, such as fountains or a Victory Horse figurine accompanied by a Ruyi, further align the energies, paving the way for prosperity and success to flow effortlessly into your life.

In 2025, the annual Flying Star 1 will influence the Southeast sector of the Luo Shu or Bagua School of Feng Shui. Traditionally associated with wealth, prosperity, and financial growth, this sector offers fertile ground for enhancing income, cash flow, and overall economic success. It brings optimism and potential for monetary advancement, making it an area ripe for strategic Feng Shui adjustments.

The Southeast is governed by the Wood element, which thrives on the nurturing qualities of Water. To amplify the financial opportunities symbolised by Flying Star 1, enhance this sector with water-themed elements such as a water feature or a picturesque water image. Water strengthens the Wood energy and harmonises with green hues, plants, and floral decorations to further support financial luck. Ensure that the water flow is directed inward, enhancing the flow of prosperity into your home rather than allowing it to exit.

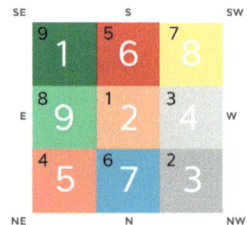

03 | MARCH
2025

The Wood Snake Year

3
Monday

Animal: **Metal Goat**
Flying Star: **5**
Good Day: **Horse**
Bad Day: **Ox**

4
Tuesday

Animal: **Water Monkey**
Flying Star: **6**
Good Day: **Snake**
Bad Day: **Tiger**

5
Wednesday

Animal: **Water Rooster**
Flying Star: **7**
Good Day: **Dragon**
Bad Day: **Rabbit**

6
Thursday

Animal: **Wood Dog**
Flying Star: **8**
Good Day: **Rabbit**
Bad Day: **Dragon**

7
Friday

Animal: **Wood Pig**
Flying Star: **9**
Good Day: **Tiger**
Bad Day: **Snake**

8
Saturday

Animal: **Fire Rat**
Flying Star: **1**
Good Day: **Ox**
Bad Day: **Horse**

9
Sunday

Animal: **Fire Ox**
Flying Star: **2**
Good Day: **Rat**
Bad Day: **Goat**

MARCH MONTHLY CHINESE ZODIAC OVERVIEW

RAT

This month calls for focus and determination. New projects will progress smoothly, but it's important to prioritise personal well-being, particularly digestive health. Address conflicts at home or work early to prevent them from escalating.

OX

Energy fluctuations will create sudden changes this month, testing your patience. Stay adaptable and manage expectations to avoid disappointment. Opportunities will come, but discernment is critical to maximising them.

TIGER

March brings fluctuating energy, so it's essential to maintain stability in your routine. Reflect on your goals and make strides towards them. Pay extra attention to personal relationships, which will require time and care.

RABBIT

This slower month is ideal for focusing on your personal needs. Avoid workplace conflicts and unnecessary changes. With weaker wealth energy, steer clear of financial risks and focus on maintaining stability.

DRAGON

This month is ideal for networking and forming new relationships. Jobseekers will benefit from sending out resumes and making connections. However, wealth energy is slow, so take a conservative approach to finances.

SNAKE

March's calm but slow energy may frustrate you, as progress will be gradual. Be cautious in communication to avoid conflict, and take extra care with money management in business and personal matters.

HORSE

If you have doubts about work, observe in the first week to find the best path forward. Emotionally, you may need a retreat to recharge. Consider a short break to refresh your mind and body.

10
Monday

Animal: **Earth Tiger**
Flying Star: **3**
Good Day: **Pig**
Bad Day: **Monkey**

11
Tuesday

Animal: **Earth Rabbit**
Flying Star: **4**
Good Day: **Dog**
Bad Day: **Rooster**

12
Wednesday

Animal: **Metal Dragon**
Flying Star: **5**
Good Day: **Rooster**
Bad Day: **Dog**

13
Thursday

Animal: **Metal Snake**
Flying Star: **6**
Good Day: **Monkey**
Bad Day: **Pig**

14
Friday

Animal: **Water Horse**
Flying Star: **7**
Good Day: **Goat**
Bad Day: **Rat**

15
Saturday

Animal: **Water Goat**
Flying Star: **8**
Good Day: **Horse**
Bad Day: **Ox**

16
Sunday

Animal: **Wood Monkey**
Flying Star: **9**
Good Day: **Snake**
Bad Day: **Tiger**

GOAT

You will feel a surge of enthusiasm this month. While progress is promising, it is important to take charge and not become complacent. Strengthen relationships with colleagues and avoid taking them for granted.

MONKEY

Positive energy continues to build, and business opportunities will flourish. If you've been considering a job change, now is the time. Relationship energy is also vital, bringing harmony to personal interactions.

ROOSTER

Mixed energy this month could bring workplace challenges due to a metaphysical clash with Rabbit. Stay patient and persistent to overcome obstacles. Financially, exercise caution and avoid impulsive spending.

DOG

March may bring unease, leading to impulses for change. Stay grounded and complete current tasks before pursuing new plans. If you have business ideas, it is best to keep them private for now.

PIG

Calm and peaceful energy reigns this month, offering a chance to assess your goals for the year. If you're considering a job change, now is the time to explore new opportunities, but wait until next month to move.

The Wood Snake Year

17
Monday

Animal: **Wood Rooster**
Flying Star: **1**
Good Day: **Dragon**
Bad Day: **Rabbit**

18
Tuesday

Animal: **Fire Dog**
Flying Star: **2**
Good Day: **Rabbit**
Bad Day: **Dragon**
✈️🏠🧧🥢🪮🎬

19
Wednesday

Animal: **Fire Pig**
Flying Star: **3**
Good Day: **Tiger**
Bad Day: **Snake**
🏠🥢🪮🎬

20
Thursday

Animal: **Earth Rat**
Flying Star: **4**
Good Day: **Ox**
Bad Day: **Horse**
👧🎗️❤️🧧

21
Friday

Animal: **Earth Ox**
Flying Star: **5**
Good Day: **Rat**
Bad Day: **Goat**
⚡🏠🧧🎬

22
Saturday

Animal: **Metal Tiger**
Flying Star: **6**
Good Day: **Pig**
Bad Day: **Monkey**
🥢🪮🎬

23
Sunday

Animal: **Metal Rabbit**
Flying Star: **7**
Good Day: **Dog**
Bad Day: **Rooster**
✈️🥢🧧🎉

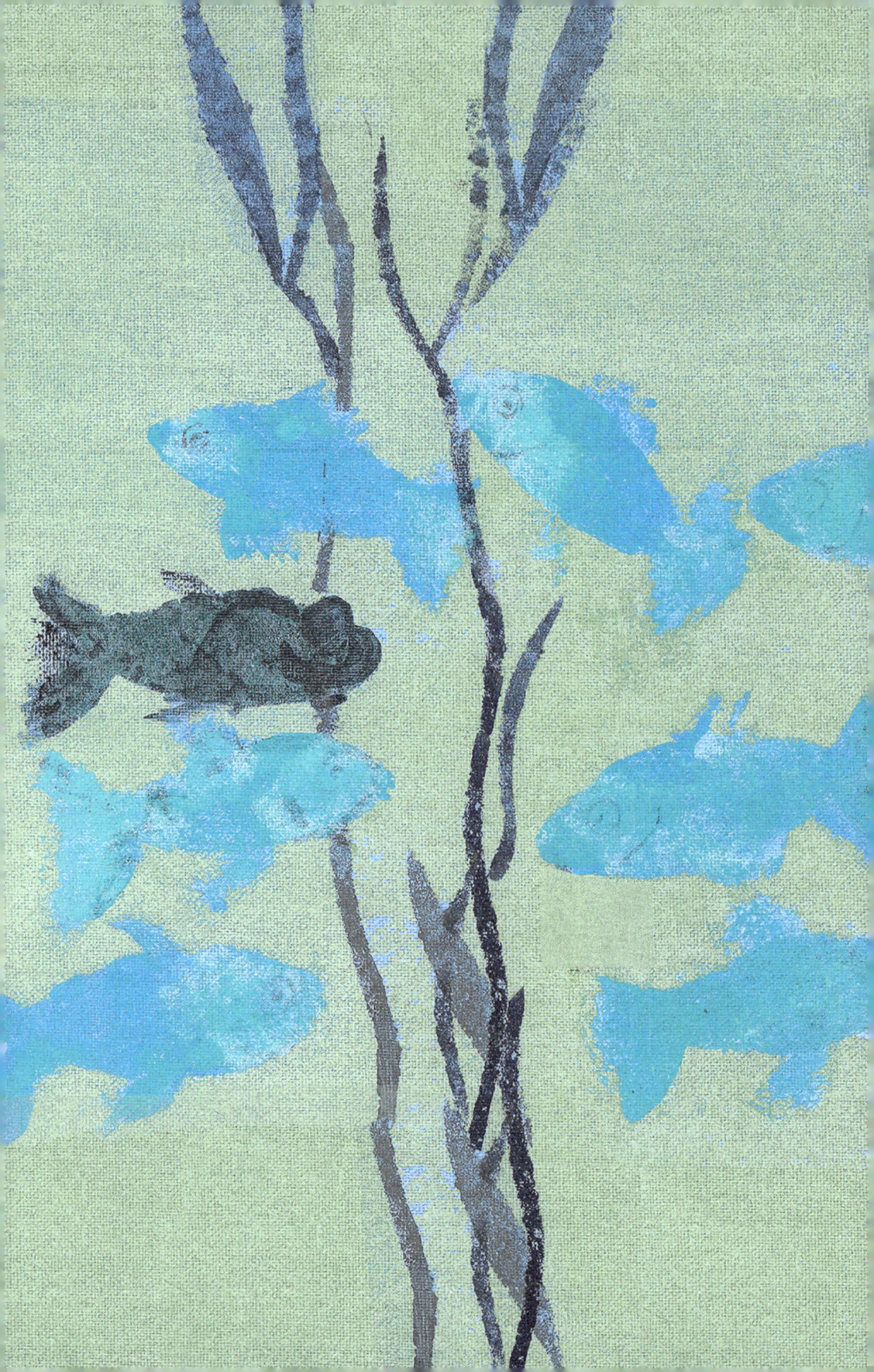

24
Monday

Animal: **Water Dragon**
Flying Star: **8**
Good Day: **Rooster**
Bad Day: **Dog**

25
Tuesday

Animal: **Water Snake**
Flying Star: **9**
Good Day: **Monkey**
Bad Day: **Pig**

26
Wednesday

Animal: **Wood Horse**
Flying Star: **1**
Good Day: **Goat**
Bad Day: **Rat**

27
Thursday

Animal: **Wood Goat**
Flying Star: **2**
Good Day: **Horse**
Bad Day: **Ox**

28
Friday

Animal: **Fire Monkey**
Flying Star: **3**
Good Day: **Snake**
Bad Day: **Tiger**

29
Saturday

Animal: **Fire Rooster**
Flying Star: **4**
Good Day: **Dragon**
Bad Day: **Rabbit**

30
Sunday

Animal: **Earth Dog**
Flying Star: **5**
Good Day: **Rabbit**
Bad Day: **Dragon**

April 5 – May 5 is the Month of the Dragon

Dragon Chinese Horoscope 2025: The Year of Transformation and Passion

Dragon Birth Years: 1916, 1928, 1940, 1952, 1964, 1976, 1988, 2000, 2012, 2024, 2036

In 2025, the Dragon will experience the dynamic and intense energies of the Yin Wood-Snake. This new influence will shift from the previous Year of the Wood Dragon, bringing transformation, passion, and heightened challenges.

Dragon-Snake Dynamic: Transformation and Challenge

The Yin Wood Snake's presence in 2025 introduces significant change and intensity. Unlike the steady growth of the Wood Dragon, the Fire Snake brings a fiery and transformative energy that may heighten emotional and professional tensions. This dynamic encourages Dragons to adapt to new circumstances and embrace change with resilience.

Elemental Influence: Wood and Fire

The Fire Snake's influence combines with the Dragon's inherent qualities, creating a potent mix of passion and transformation. While the previous year's Wood element fostered growth and innovation, the Fire Snake's energy emphasises personal and professional upheavals. This year will require Dragons to effectively manage intense emotions and harness their transformative power.

Harnessing Passion and Transformation

The vibrant and intense nature of the Fire Snake demands that Dragons balance their ambitious goals with emotional intelligence. Embracing this fiery energy can lead to profound personal and professional breakthroughs, but it also requires careful management of stress and conflict.

Love Horoscope: Intensity and Growth

In matters of the heart, the Year of the Yin Wood Snake brings excitement and challenges. Relationships may experience intense emotions and transformative shifts. For single Dragons, the year is ripe for passionate encounters, though maintaining patience and communication is crucial. Those in committed relationships must navigate heightened emotions and focus on deepening their bonds.

Career Horoscope: Innovation and Adaptation

The Fire Snake's transformative energy characterises career prospects in 2025. Dragons may face significant shifts and opportunities that require adaptability and strategic thinking. Embrace innovation and be prepared for sudden changes. Fields that thrive on creativity and adaptability, such as tech and entertainment, will be particularly favourable.

Finance Horoscope: Caution and Opportunity

The financial landscape for Dragons in 2025 will be marked by both risk and reward. The Fire Snake's influence calls for careful planning and risk assessment. Avoid impulsive financial decisions and focus on strategic investments—research before committing to new ventures to capitalise on emerging opportunities while minimising potential losses.

Health Horoscope: Balance and Wellness

Maintaining health and well-being is essential amid the Fire Snake's intense energy. Dragons should prioritise a balanced lifestyle, including regular exercise, adequate rest, and stress management techniques. The year's transformative energy can be harnessed to enhance overall vitality and resilience, but avoiding burnout is crucial.

Dragon and Snake Partnership: Growth and Challenge

The interplay between the Dragon's power and the Snake's intensity creates a year of significant change and potential growth. Dragons must navigate the Snake's passionate energy with strategic foresight and emotional balance. They must embrace transformative opportunities while managing challenges with diplomacy and adaptability.

Holistic Prosperity: Embracing Transformation

The Year of the Yin Wood Snake offers profound opportunities for growth and transformation. While the energy may bring challenges, it also paves the way for significant personal and professional achievements. Balance passion with practicality to achieve a successful and fulfilling year.

Health and Vitality: Mindful Practices

With the Fire Snake's dynamic influence, maintaining health requires a mindful approach. Incorporate regular exercise, meditation, and balanced nutrition to manage stress and support overall well-being. The intensity of the year necessitates a proactive approach to health.

Dragon and Snake Synergy: Success and Adaptation

Combining the Dragon's inherent strength and the Snake's transformative energy sets the stage for a year of significant achievement and adaptation. By embracing the intensity and navigating the challenges with resilience, Dragons can achieve substantial success and personal growth.

Chinese Zodiac Dragon: Embracing the Fire Snake's Energy

The transition from the Wood Dragon to the Yin Wood Snake marks a year of intense change and opportunity. Dragons are encouraged to adapt to the transformative energy, balance passion with practicality, and leverage the year's dynamics to achieve personal and professional success.

2025: Dragon and Snake Synergy

The collaboration between the Dragon and the Fire Snake introduces a period of growth, passion, and transformation. Embrace the challenges and opportunities this dynamic year presents to achieve a successful and transformative year ahead.

APRIL Flying Star 9: Abundant Prosperity and Beyond

April rejoices under the luminous influence of Flying Star 9, a radiant beacon in the celestial tapestry. Known as the Star of Current Prosperity, this star shines brilliantly over completion, fame, celebration, wealth, intelligence, popularity, happiness, and acclaim. As a dynamic Fire Star, its vibrant energy sparks a cascade of joyous gatherings and festive occasions, inviting all to bask in its auspicious glow. Dubbed the "Star of Completion," Flying Star 9 brings projects and endeavours to their triumphant conclusion, nurturing financial success and prosperity.

This star is a powerful catalyst for both present and future ventures, magnifying the means of abundance and ensuring that previously sown seeds of effort bear fruit. Its influence is particularly potent for the eldest son and those born under the Rabbit sign, as Flying Star 9 illuminates their paths with its brilliant energy.

As the ultimate harbinger of prosperity, Flying Star 9 accelerates wealth accumulation, boosts business profits, and enhances investments. It also elevates fame and recognition, casting a celestial spotlight on those pursuing success in various fields. In the current cosmic configuration, Flying Star 9 is the most potent force among divine energies, making engaging with spaces influenced by this star highly beneficial. Whether embarking on new business ventures, planning a wedding, or starting a family, the energy of Flying Star 9 offers a powerful boost to these life-changing endeavours.

To amplify its auspicious energy, incorporate wealth-enhancing symbols into your surroundings. Consider placing a wealth jar, Buddha figurines, or a trio of horses in prominent positions. Arranging 9 Gold Coins on a tassel or displaying a Wealth God figure and Gold Ingots further strengthens the star's influence. Multiples of nine, vibrant lighting, and red-themed decor—such as red phoenix symbols, upholstery, and accessories—elevate the energy even more. For an extra touch of prosperity, introduce a water feature with nine fish to amplify the flow of abundance.

Flying Star 9 emerges as a radiant symbol of prosperity and joy, guiding all who embrace its effervescent energy toward a bountiful journey ahead.

In 2025, the East sector of the Luo Shu or Bagua School of Feng Shui will be graced by the annual Flying Star 9. This sector, deeply associated with health, longevity, and overall well-being, provides a prime opportunity to enhance these vital aspects of life.

The Wood element governs the East, and incorporating both Wood and Water elements can amplify its positive influence on health and vitality. One effective remedy is to place bamboo in a water feature, as this combination strengthens the Wood element and supports a flourishing state of health. Introducing greenery, plants, and vibrant flowers will further invigorate this sector. The East is also home to the celestial Green Dragon, a symbol of auspicious fortune. Positioning a dragon figurine in this area can optimise the family's luck and overall well-being. Consider placing a Quan Yin statue to safeguard and nurture your physical and emotional vitality for added protection and health enhancement.

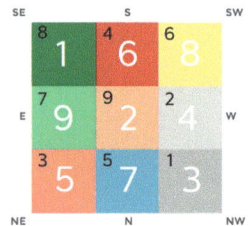

SE	S	SW
8 **1**	4 **6**	6 **8**
7 **9**	9 **2**	2 **4**
3 **5**	5 **7**	1 **3**
NE	N	NW

31
Monday

Animal: **Earth Pig**
Flying Star: **6**
Good Day: **Tiger**
Bad Day: **Snake**

1
Tuesday

Animal: **Metal Rat**
Flying Star: **7**
Good Day: **Ox**
Bad Day: **Horse**

2
Wednesday

Animal: **Metal Ox**
Flying Star: **8**
Good Day: **Rat**
Bad Day: **Goat**

3
Thursday

Animal: **Water Tiger**
Flying Star: **9**
Good Day: **Pig**
Bad Day: **Monkey**

4
Friday

Animal: **Water Rabbit**
Flying Star: **1**
Good Day: **Dog**
Bad Day: **Rooster**

5
Saturday

Animal: **Wood Dragon**
Flying Star: **2**
Good Day: **Rooster**
Bad Day: **Dog**

6
Sunday

Animal: **Wood Snake**
Flying Star: **3**
Good Day: **Monkey**
Bad Day: **Pig**

APRIL MONTHLY CHINESE ZODIAC OVERVIEW

RAT

Energy fluctuations this month may cause restlessness, so avoid rushing decisions. Be thorough with your work, especially when sharing information. Address conflicts early and ensure you are not underselling yourself in negotiations. Engage in outdoor activities to relieve stress and clear your mind.

OX

April may feel emotionally draining. Stay balanced and attentive to your health while avoiding procrastination in business matters. Trust your intuition and make firm decisions to stay ahead. Avoid misleading influences, and be proactive in managing your well-being.

TIGER

April may test your patience with restless energy. Rather than rushing ahead, focus on what's right in front of you. Business owners should remain open to new ideas, and travel may be on the horizon. Slow down to embrace opportunities for personal growth.

RABBIT

April could bring emotional sensitivity. If conflicts arise at home, resolve them quickly. At work, remain optimistic and focus on completing tasks. Avoid hasty decisions, especially financial ones, to prevent mistakes.

DRAGON

As positive energy builds, you'll feel empowered this month. Work will gain momentum, and new ventures will be favoured. Financial power is emphasised, but outcomes may vary, so manage resources carefully and avoid unnecessary risks.

SNAKE

Energy shifts this month are bringing smoother progress at work. People will be more helpful, so remain open to new connections and opportunities. Financial energy is slow, so avoid overspending. A short vacation will be beneficial for recharging.

HORSE

Business will improve by mid-month, but maintain a cheerful mindset. Suppose you are considering a new business venture; thoroughly research before diving in. Be mindful of your health and make time for self-care to balance your workload.

The Wood Snake Year

7
Monday

Animal: **Fire Horse**
Flying Star: **4**
Good Day: **Goat**
Bad Day: **Rat**
✈️ 🐒 ❤️ 🗞️ 🥢 🎉

8
Tuesday

Animal: **Fire Goat**
Flying Star: **5**
Good Day: **Horse**
Bad Day: **Ox**
⚡

9
Wednesday

Animal: **Earth Monkey**
Flying Star: **6**
Good Day: **Snake**
Bad Day: **Tiger**
👞🏭

10
Thursday

Animal: **Earth Rooster**
Flying Star: **7**
Good Day: **Dragon**
Bad Day: **Rabbit**

11
Friday

Animal: **Metal Dog**
Flying Star: **8**
Good Day: **Rabbit**
Bad Day: **Dragon**

12
Saturday

Animal: **Metal Pig**
Flying Star: **9**
Good Day: **Tiger**
Bad Day: **Snake**

13
Sunday

Animal: **Water Rat**
Flying Star: **1**
Good Day: **Ox**
Bad Day: **Horse**
🏭

GOAT

April will bring business delays, so it's crucial to protect your personal and business information. Financial energy is slow, so exercise caution with large transactions. Stay focused and patient while navigating the month's obstacles.

MONKEY

Positive energy continues to build, and the business is likely to thrive. Clear communication is essential to avoid misunderstandings, and patience will be vital for managing projects effectively. Stay proactive, and success will follow.

ROOSTER

April's unstable energy requires patience. With thoughtful planning, you will find support and make progress. Wealth energy fluctuates, so avoid major financial moves and focus on careful, conservative approaches.

DOG

April's unpredictable energy calls for flexibility. While work may not progress as planned, persistence will pay off. Spend time with supportive people and focus on decluttering your space to shift stagnant energy.

PIG

April offers robust and supportive energy. It's a great time for positive steps in work and personal life. Thorough preparation is vital if you're planning new ventures. Focus on well-being and balanced living to thrive.

The Wood Snake Year

14
Monday

Animal: **Water Ox**
Flying Star: **2**
Good Day: **Rat**
Bad Day: **Goat**

15
Tuesday

Animal: **Wood Tiger**
Flying Star: **3**
Good Day: **Pig**
Bad Day: **Monkey**
🏠🐚✂️ ✈️ 🎆🎬

16
Wednesday

Animal: **Wood Rabbit**
Flying Star: **4**
Good Day: **Dog**
Bad Day: **Rooster**
❤️👙🥢✂️🎬

17
Thursday

Animal: **Fire Dragon**
Flying Star: **5**
Good Day: **Rooster**
Bad Day: **Dog**
⚡✈️

18
Friday

Animal: **Fire Snake**
Flying Star: **6**
Good Day: **Monkey**
Bad Day: **Pig**

19
Saturday

Animal: **Earth Horse**
Flying Star: **7**
Good Day: **Goat**
Bad Day: **Rat**
✈️🐿️🥢🐚🎆

20
Sunday

Animal: **Earth Goat**
Flying Star: **8**
Good Day: **Horse**
Bad Day: **Ox**

FENG SHUI PRINCIPLES FOR THE BEDROOM

The feng shui in your bedroom is of utmost importance, given that it's where you spend your most vulnerable and restorative hours. Tailoring feng shui principles to your style can enhance the overall energy and luck in your bedroom's decor.

Essential General Tips for the Bedroom:

Ensure your bedroom is of regular shape without missing corners for balanced energy flow.

Keep plants and flowers out of the bedroom, as they can drain your energy, leaving you fatigued despite a good night's sleep.

Choose a bed that is the right size for you; one that is too small may hinder personal growth, while an overly large bed can contribute to relationship issues.

Opt for bedroom furniture with rounded edges and corners, avoiding overly angular designs to prevent the formation of harmful poison arrows that may lead to serious illness if left uncorrected.

Position the bed with the headboard against a wall, avoiding a "floating" arrangement in the centre of the bedroom.

Orient your bed to one of your auspicious directions for a more harmonious sleeping experience.

Minimise or avoid mirrors in the bedroom; place them inside a cabinet if necessary. Ensure that mirrors, especially on dressing tables, do not directly face the bed, as exposed mirrors may invite interference in your relationships.

Choose neutral and relaxing colours for the bedroom to maintain a balanced energy. Avoid excessive Yang energy, which disrupts sleep patterns and keeps you awake at night.

The Wood Snake Year

21 Monday

Animal: **Metal Monkey**
Flying Star: **9**
Good Day: **Snake**
Bad Day: **Tiger**

22 Tuesday

Animal: **Metal Rooster**
Flying Star: **1**
Good Day: **Dragon**
Bad Day: **Rabbit**

23 Wednesday

Animal: **Water Dog**
Flying Star: **2**
Good Day: **Rabbit**
Bad Day: **Dragon**

24 Thursday

Animal: **Water Pig**
Flying Star: **3**
Good Day: **Tiger**
Bad Day: **Snake**

25 Friday

Animal: **Wood Rat**
Flying Star: **4**
Good Day: **Ox**
Bad Day: **Horse**

26 Saturday

Animal: **Wood Ox**
Flying Star: **5**
Good Day: **Rat**
Bad Day: **Goat**

27 Sunday

Animal: **Fire Tiger**
Flying Star: **6**
Good Day: **Pig**
Bad Day: **Monkey**

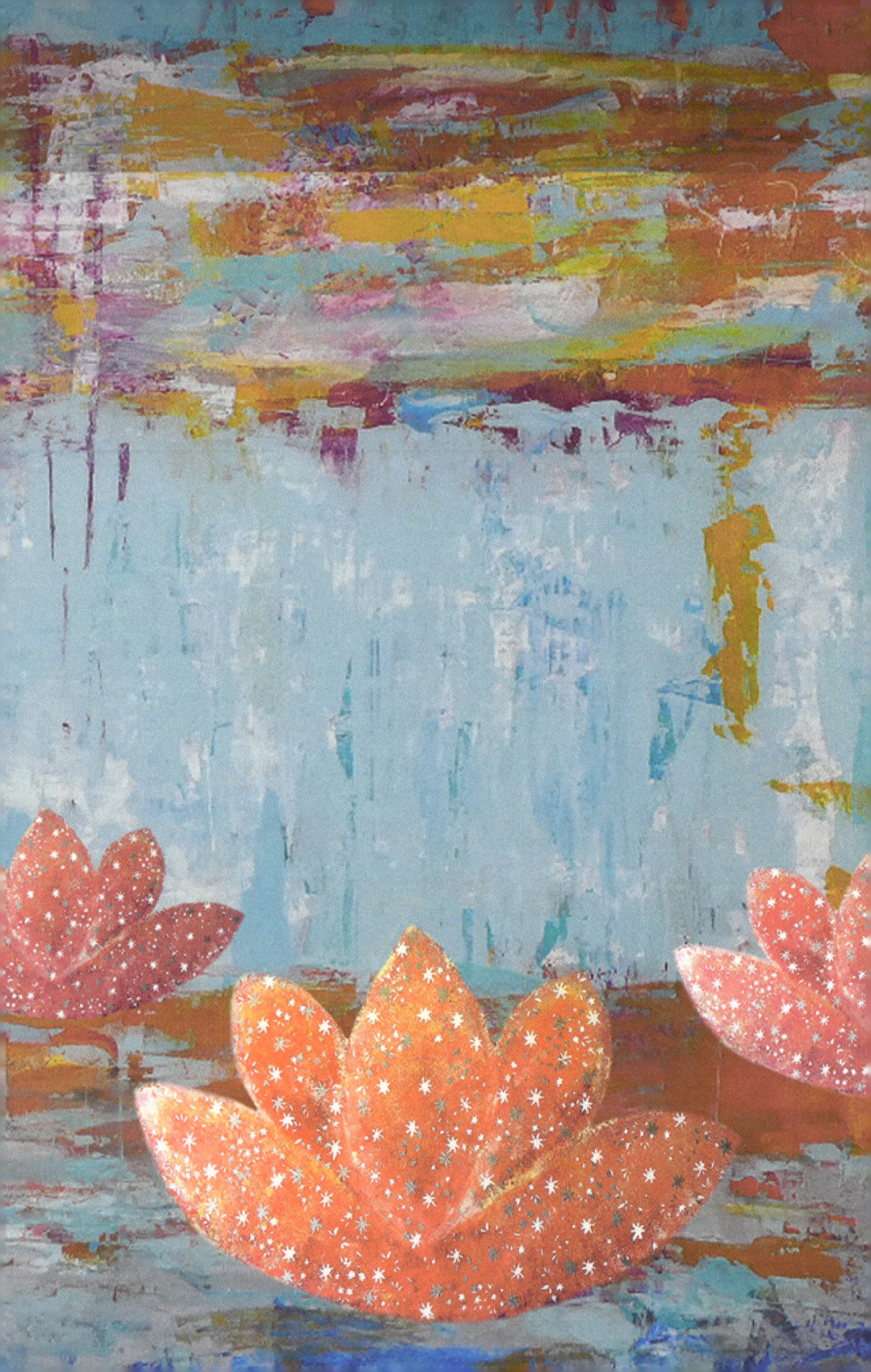

The Wood Snake Year

28
Monday

Animal: **Fire Rabbit**
Flying Star: **7**
Good Day: **Dog**
Bad Day: **Rooster**
✈️🎰

29
Tuesday

Animal: **Earth Dragon**
Flying Star: **8**
Good Day: **Rooster**
Bad Day: **Dog**

30
Wednesday

Animal: **Earth Snake**
Flying Star: **9**
Good Day: **Monkey**
Bad Day: **Pig**
🏠💿

1
Thursday

Animal: **Metal Horse**
Flying Star: **1**
Good Day: **Goat**
Bad Day: **Rat**
✈️💿🎉

2
Friday

Animal: **Metal Goat**
Flying Star: **2**
Good Day: **Horse**
Bad Day: **Ox**

3
Saturday

Animal: **Water Monkey**
Flying Star: **3**
Good Day: **Snake**
Bad Day: **Tiger**
🎰

4
Sunday

Animal: **Water Rooster**
Flying Star: **4**
Good Day: **Dragon**
Bad Day: **Rabbit**
🐟❤️✈️

May 6 – June 5 is the Month of the Snake

Snake Chinese Horoscope 2025: Navigating Passion and Transformation

Snake Birth Years: 1917, 1929, 1941, 1953, 1965, 1977, 1989, 2001, 2013, 2025, 2037

In 2025, the Snake will encounter the vibrant and intense energies of the Yin Wood-Snake. This year introduces a shift from the previous Wood Dragon influence, focusing on passion, transformation, and adaptability.

Snake-Fire Snake Dynamic: Passion and Transformation

With the Year of the Yin Wood Snake, the Snake experiences a period of heightened intensity and change. This year's energy emphasises profound personal and professional transformation and passionate and potentially tumultuous experiences. Adapting to these changes with flexibility and resilience will be crucial for success.

Elemental Influence: Wood and Fire

The Fire Snake's influence in 2025 introduces a fiery and dynamic energy that contrasts with the previous year's steady growth. While Wood represents growth and creativity, the Fire element ignites transformation and intensity. This combination demands that Snakes harness their passion effectively while navigating the challenges of a transformative year.

Career and Professional Growth: Embracing Change

In 2025, Snakes will face significant opportunities for career growth and transformation. The intense Fire Snake energy encourages Snakes to step out of their comfort zones, embrace new challenges, and pursue innovative projects. Fields that involve creativity, leadership, and adaptability will see the most success. Staying open to change and developing new skills will enhance career prospects.

Financial Outlook: Opportunities and Caution

Potential gains and risks will mark the financial landscape for Snakes in 2025. The Fire Snake's volatile energy requires careful financial planning and risk management. Invest wisely in sectors that align with your goals, and avoid impulsive decisions. Thorough research and strategic investments will lead to economic stability and growth.

Love and Relationships: Intensity and Communication

The Year of the Yin Wood Snake brings a passionate and intense energy to love and relationships. Snakes may experience profound emotional shifts and transformative encounters. Effective communication, patience, and openness are essential to navigate potential challenges. For singles, new and exciting connections are possible, while those in relationships should focus on deepening their bonds and managing heightened emotions.

Health and Wellness: Balancing Intensity

Maintaining health and well-being is crucial amid the intense energy of the Fire Snake. Snakes should prioritise self-care, including regular exercise, stress management, and a balanced lifestyle. The year's transformative energy can lead to physical and emotional fatigue, so adapting to changes and practising mindfulness is essential to sustain overall vitality.

Symbolism of the Snake: Passion and Transformation

In 2025, the Snake symbolises passion, transformation, and adaptability. The Fire Snake's influence brings intense personal and professional growth. Embrace this transformative energy with an open mind and strategic approach to navigate the challenges and opportunities that arise.

2025: A Year of Intensity and Growth

The Year of the Yin Wood Snake offers a unique blend of passion and transformation. Snakes can achieve significant personal and professional growth by harnessing the year's dynamic energy and remaining adaptable. Embrace change with resilience and strategic foresight to make the most of the opportunities that 2025 presents.

MAY, Flying Star 8: Unveiling Abundant Prosperity

May usher in a steady wave of prosperity with the presence of the retiring Flying Star 8. Within the grand celestial orchestra, this star shines brilliantly as the Star of Prosperity, casting an encompassing glow of wealth, well-being, luxury, renown, financial prowess, and lasting success. Flying Star 8 is a beacon of affluence, bringing monetary fortune, nobility, and enduring stability. Under its benevolent light, one can anticipate an increase in income, financial triumphs, and the fortunate alignment of power and influence. As its radiant energy resonates, professional pursuits flourish, enhancing reputation and recognition for hard work. To align with this favourable tide is to unlock a world of growing potential.

For homes with a Southwest-facing main door or a living or family area in this sector, Flying Star 8's optimistic energy becomes an all-encompassing blessing. Particularly advantageous for matriarchs, mothers, older women, and those born under the Goat or Monkey zodiac signs, this star's influence extends with generosity and grace.

Maintaining a clutter-free space in this sector ensures a smooth energy flow. To activate and amplify its auspicious vibrations, incorporating wealth-related symbols serves as a powerful enhancer. These symbols might include a Buddha figurine, a tassel adorned with 6 Gold Coins, a Wealth God figure, or Gold Ingots. Additionally, the strategic placement of bright lights, clocks, and televisions, along with fostering an environment bustling with activity, significantly boosts the star's positive influence. Notably, movement—whether through footsteps or other dynamic actions—remains the most potent conductor of energy in this space.

Flying Star 8's brilliance unveils a realm of luxury and affluence. To embrace its blessings is to enter a world of enduring prosperity and unyielding success.

In 2025, the Southwest sector of the Luo Shu or Bagua School of Feng Shui will host the annual Flying Star 8. This sector is pivotal for fostering relationship luck, love, romance, and marriage, making it a vital area for enhancing these aspects of life.

The Southwest is associated with the Earth element, and to amplify its positive effects on relationships, integrating both Earth and Fire energies is critical. Enhance this sector with amethyst or rose quartz crystals, and consider incorporating vibrant hues such as purple, pink, and red peonies to support romantic endeavours. The double happiness symbol and a pair of Mandarin Ducks are traditional symbols that signify love and partnership, making them ideal for this area. To further boost the energy, add bright lighting to the Southwest sector, illuminating it with positive and nurturing vibrations.

05 | MAY 2025

The Wood Snake Year

5
Monday

Animal: **Wood Dog**
Flying Star: **5**
Good Day: **Rabbit**
Bad Day: **Dragon**
⚡✈️🎬

6
Tuesday

Animal: **Wood Pig**
Flying Star: **6**
Good Day: **Tiger**
Bad Day: **Snake**

7
Wednesday

Animal: **Fire Rat**
Flying Star: **7**
Good Day: **Ox**
Bad Day: **Horse**
🏠✈️👟🎬

8
Thursday

Animal: **Fire Ox**
Flying Star: **8**
Good Day: **Rat**
Bad Day: **Goat**
👟🎬

9
Friday

Animal: **Earth Tiger**
Flying Star: **9**
Good Day: **Pig**
Bad Day: **Monkey**

10
Saturday

Animal: **Earth Rabbit**
Flying Star: **1**
Good Day: **Dog**
Bad Day: **Rooster**
✈️👟

11
Sunday

Animal: **Metal Dragon**
Flying Star: **2**
Good Day: **Rooster**
Bad Day: **Dog**
✈️🏠👟🎬

MAY MONTHLY CHINESE ZODIAC OVERVIEW

RAT

This is one of your best months of the year, filled with positive energy. New business ventures and collaborations will succeed. Wealth energy is vital, but be cautious of overspending. Harmonious relationships make this a peaceful month.

OX

It may bring relationship stress, so remain calm and grounded. Hold your position until things stabilise, especially in a new business or job. Stay steady, and this challenging period will pass.

TIGER

Old issues may resurface for healing, but this is an opportunity for growth. Financial energy is positive, but avoid partnerships this month. Relationships will improve, so treat yourself and others with care and compassion.

RABBIT

It may present some energetic challenges, so practicality is essential. Be mindful of your finances and avoid taking on new debt. While wealth energy is weaker, other aspects of your life will remain peaceful and stable.

DRAGON

This may bring uncertainties, leading to concern. Focus on the positive aspects of life and take advantage of early-month solid financial energy. Prioritise your safety and well-being to prevent potential harm.

SNAKE

As a clashing month, avoid creating problems by keeping a low profile. Refrain from big decisions and be cautious of triggering adverse incidents that could have long-lasting effects. Stick to a conservative approach.

HORSE

May's energy is progressive, and many of your plans will come to fruition. Review your dreams and goals, reflecting on how far you've come. This is an excellent time to gain clarity on the future.

The Wood Snake Year

12
Monday

Animal: **Metal Snake**
Flying Star: **3**
Good Day: **Monkey**
Bad Day: **Pig**

13
Tuesday

Animal: **Water Horse**
Flying Star: **4**
Good Day: **Goat**
Bad Day: **Rat**

14
Wednesday

Animal: **Water Goat**
Flying Star: **5**
Good Day: **Horse**
Bad Day: **Ox**

15
Thursday

Animal: **Wood Monkey**
Flying Star: **6**
Good Day: **Snake**
Bad Day: **Tiger**

16
Friday

Animal: **Wood Rooster**
Flying Star: **7**
Good Day: **Dragon**
Bad Day: **Rabbit**

17
Saturday

Animal: **Fire Dog**
Flying Star: **8**
Good Day: **Rabbit**
Bad Day: **Dragon**

18
Sunday

Animal: **Fire Pig**
Flying Star: **9**
Good Day: **Tiger**
Bad Day: **Snake**

GOAT

May will be exceptionally busy, with some projects taking longer than expected. Service industries may experience stress due to understaffing. Financial energy is stable, but careful management is advised to avoid issues.

MONKEY

May brings clarity and optimism with new opportunities for advancement. Creative energy will flow, leading to innovative ideas and business success. Stay adaptable and proactive to capitalise on this promising period.

ROOSTER

A surge of positive energy will empower you this month, making it a great time to implement your plans. Business prospects look strong, and expansion is possible. Embrace changes confidently.

DOG

Calm energy will support your progress this month. You'll be enthusiastic about new ideas, and financially, opportunities for gains are substantial. Socially, this is a vibrant time filled with interesting new connections.

PIG

May's clashing energy could bring fluctuations, so proceed cautiously. If possible, take time for self-care and a vacation. Stay patient and avoid unnecessary risks to maintain stability.

19
Monday

Animal: **Earth Rat**
Flying Star: **1**
Good Day: **Ox**
Bad Day: **Horse**

20
Tuesday

Animal: **Earth Ox**
Flying Star: **2**
Good Day: **Rat**
Bad Day: **Goat**

21
Wednesday

Animal: **Metal Tiger**
Flying Star: **3**
Good Day: **Pig**
Bad Day: **Monkey**

22
Thursday

Animal: **Metal Rabbit**
Flying Star: **4**
Good Day: **Dog**
Bad Day: **Rooster**

23
Friday

Animal: **Water Dragon**
Flying Star: **5**
Good Day: **Rooster**
Bad Day: **Dog**

24
Saturday

Animal: **Water Snake**
Flying Star: **6**
Good Day: **Monkey**
Bad Day: **Pig**

25
Sunday

Animal: **Wood Horse**
Flying Star: **7**
Good Day: **Goat**
Bad Day: **Rat**

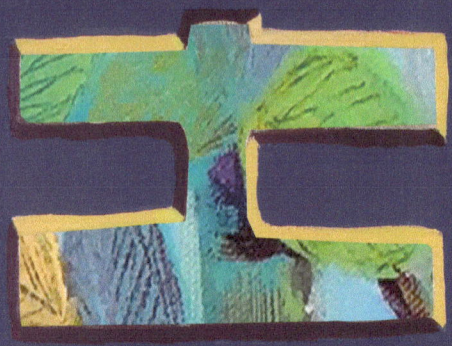

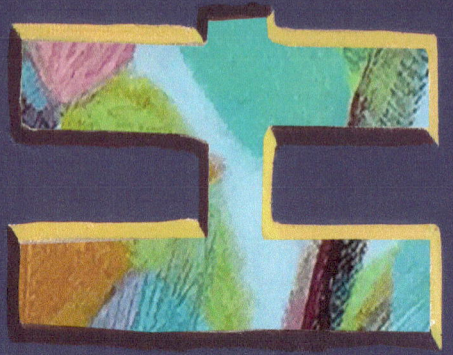

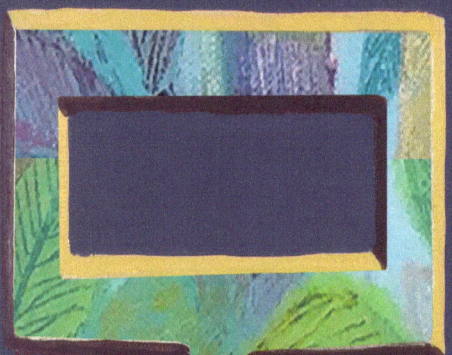

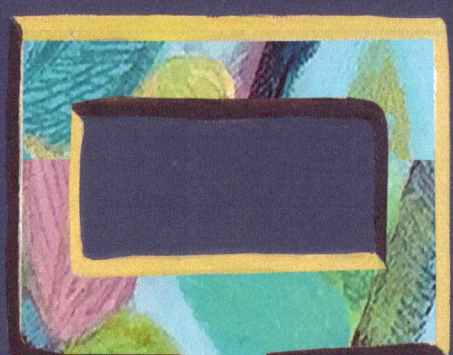

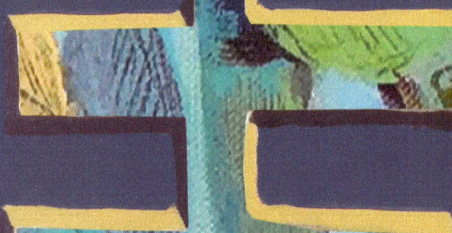

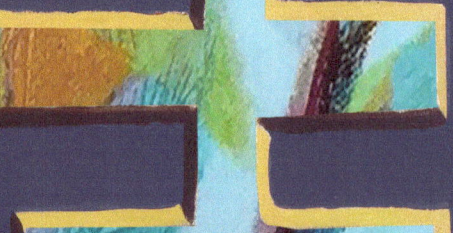

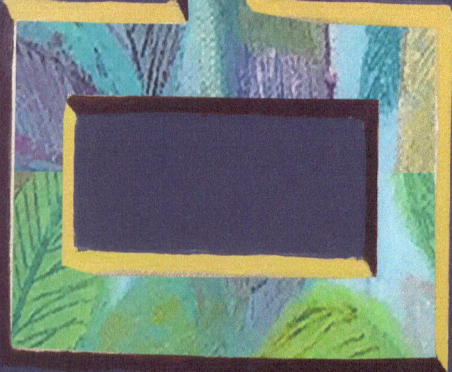

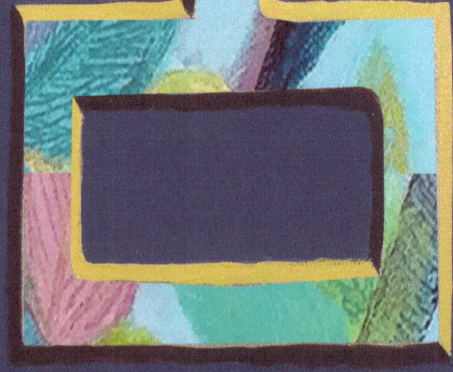

The Wood Snake Year

26
Monday

Animal: **Wood Goat**
Flying Star: **8**
Good Day: **Horse**
Bad Day: **Ox**

27
Tuesday

Animal: **Fire Monkey**
Flying Star: **9**
Good Day: **Snake**
Bad Day: **Tiger**

28
Wednesday

Animal: **Fire Rooster**
Flying Star: **1**
Good Day: **Dragon**
Bad Day: **Rabbit**

29
Thursday

Animal: **Earth Dog**
Flying Star: **2**
Good Day: **Rabbit**
Bad Day: **Dragon**

30
Friday

Animal: **Earth Pig**
Flying Star: **3**
Good Day: **Tiger**
Bad Day: **Snake**

31
Saturday

Animal: **Metal Rat**
Flying Star: **4**
Good Day: **Ox**
Bad Day: **Horse**

1
Sunday

Animal: **Metal Ox**
Flying Star: **5**
Good Day: **Rat**
Bad Day: **Goat**

June 6 – July 6 is the Month of the Horse

Horse Chinese Horoscope 2025: Embracing Passion and Adaptability

Horse Birth Years: **1918, 1930, 1942, 1954, 1966, 1978, 1990, 2002, 2014, 2026, 2038**

In 2025, the Horse will experience the dynamic and passionate energies of the Yin Wood-Snake. This year brings an energetic shift from the previous Year of the Wood Dragon, emphasising transformation, passion, and adaptability.

Fire Snake Influence: Passion and Transformation

The Year of the Yin Wood Snake introduces a period of heightened passion and transformation for the Horse. This fiery energy contrasts the previous year's steadiness, bringing opportunities and challenges. Horses must adapt quickly and harness their inherent dynamism to thrive in this vibrant environment.

Career and Professional Opportunities: Seizing the Moment

In 2025, Horses will encounter exciting career opportunities fuelled by the Fire Snake's influence. This year favours bold moves and innovative thinking. Horses are encouraged to embrace change, take calculated risks, and pursue new ventures. Adaptability and creativity will be vital to navigating the challenges and maximising emerging opportunities.

Financial Outlook: Caution and Strategic Investments

Financially, the Year of the Fire Snake presents potential gains and risks. The intense and unpredictable nature of the Fire Snake calls for careful financial planning and strategic investments. Horses should approach investments with caution and avoid impulsive decisions. Conduct thorough research and focus on opportunities that align with long-term goals.

Love and Relationships: Intensity and Communication

The Fire Snake's passionate energy brings a dynamic shift to love and relationships. For single Horses, this year offers the possibility of intense and transformative connections. Patience and clear communication are essential for building trust and navigating potential challenges. Committed Horses may experience heightened emotions, requiring open dialogue and understanding to strengthen relationships.

Career Challenges and Growth: Embracing Change

Both opportunities and obstacles will mark the career landscape for Horses in 2025. The Fire Snake's influence encourages Horses to embrace change and pursue new professional paths. While there may be challenges, particularly in adapting to new roles or projects, the year's energetic drive offers significant growth and achievement potential.

Wealth and Investment: Strategic Planning

Financially, Horses will need to be strategic and cautious. The Fire Snake's volatile nature necessitates careful planning and risk management. Focus on stable and promising investment opportunities while avoiding high-risk ventures. Leveraging creativity and adaptability will help you navigate the financial landscape effectively.

Health and Wellness: Balancing Intensity

With the intense energy of the Fire Snake, maintaining health and wellness is crucial. Horses should prioritise a balanced lifestyle, incorporating regular exercise, stress management, and healthy eating habits. The year's dynamic energy may lead to physical and emotional fatigue, so adapting and practising self-care is essential to sustain overall well-being.

Symbolism of the Horse and Fire Snake: Passion and Transformation

In 2025, the Horse's inherent drive and the Fire Snake's transformative energy create a powerful combination. This year symbolises a period of intense personal and professional growth. By harnessing the Fire Snake's passion and staying adaptable, Horses can navigate challenges and seize opportunities for success.

2025: A Year of Dynamic Growth and Adaptability

The Year of the Yin Wood Snake offers the Horse a vibrant and transformative experience. Embracing change, leveraging passion, and maintaining strategic focus will be essential for thriving in this energetic year. By adapting to the Fire Snake's dynamic influence, Horses can achieve significant growth and success.

JUNE, Flying Star 7: A Multitude of Discord and Unrest

June heralds a period of unrest with the arrival of the ominous Flying Star 7. In the intricate cosmic dance, this inauspicious star ushers in a cacophony of conflict, disputes, legal entanglements, ailments, mishaps, theft, and the unsettling echoes of gossip. The shadow cast by Flying Star 7 is profoundly feared, as it has the potential to sow seeds of rivalry, trespass, theft, and even violence into the fabric of life. During this phase, caution is essential, as one must carefully navigate its treacherous currents.

The unsettling energies of this star are particularly potent in matters of emotional and physical well-being, making vigilance crucial for those in the middle son or middle-aged man category or those born under the Rat zodiac sign. In professional environments, office politics swell, and rivalries intensify. Trust must be earned as deception and schemes lurk beneath the surface. The South sector, in particular, resonates with this turbulence, and therefore, heightened awareness and vigilance are vital to maintaining tranquillity.

Flying Star 7 also brings the risk of ailments related to the mouth and teeth, potentially leading to the need for hospitalisation or surgical interventions for those with pre-existing health issues. Traditional remedies become essential in mitigating its disruptive influence. One such remedy involves placing three pieces of bamboo in a clear glass vase filled with water in the Western sector. The symbolic talisman of the Evil Eye, flanked by seven glass elephants, serves as a powerful countermeasure. Positioning a Blue Rhinoceros and a Blue Elephant can protect against this evil energy. As a final safeguard, incorporating a water feature helps to neutralise the metallic energy dominating this space, ensuring the tranquillity and vitality of the surrounding environment.

Flying Star 7's arrival necessitates a mindful approach, as its discordant energies require careful navigation to avoid being swept into its currents of unrest and discord.

In 2025, the North sector of the Luo Shu or Bagua School of Feng Shui will be graced by the annual Flying Star 7, a key influence on career and business fortune.

The Water element governs the North, and to bolster this sector for optimal career and business success, it is essential to harmonise the Water energy with Metal elements. Enhance the North with metallic colours such as white, silver, gold, pewter, bronze, and black tones to support and balance the Water energy. Incorporate metal décor objects with blue-black accents, and consider adding water-themed pictures or decorative elements to amplify the positive influence. Additionally, placing a Black Tortoise or Dragon Tortoise in this area can further strengthen career prospects and business growth.

The Wood Snake Year

2 Monday	Animal: **Water Tiger** Flying Star: **6** Good Day: **Pig** Bad Day: **Monkey**
3 Tuesday	Animal: **Water Rabbit** Flying Star: **7** Good Day: **Dog** Bad Day: **Rooster**
4 Wednesday	Animal: **Wood Dragon** Flying Star: **8** Good Day: **Rooster** Bad Day: **Dog**
5 Thursday	Animal: **Wood Snake** Flying Star: **9** Good Day: **Monkey** Bad Day: **Pig**
6 Friday	Animal: **Fire Horse** Flying Star: **1** Good Day: **Goat** Bad Day: **Rat**
7 Saturday	Animal: **Fire Goat** Flying Star: **2** Good Day: **Horse** Bad Day: **Ox**
8 Sunday	Animal: **Earth Monkey** Flying Star: **3** Good Day: **Snake** Bad Day: **Tiger**

JUNE MONTHLY CHINESE ZODIAC OVERVIEW

RAT

June may bring irritability, so take time to relax and maintain balance. Real estate dealings will be rewarding. Pay close attention to health, especially heart and blood-related concerns, and prioritise a healthy lifestyle.

OX

June is one of the best months for business planning and project initiation. While significant changes to work systems aren't recommended, financial energy is vital for increasing income and profits.

TIGER

Enjoyable and exciting energy fills June with financial gains from sales or investments. Job changes and new business opportunities are favourable. Real estate dealings are also promising, making this a productive month.

RABBIT

June's improved energy creates a favourable environment for work and business. Networking will bring powerful connections, so treat yourself with kindness and focus on health. Financial energy stabilises mid-month.

DRAGON

Small emotional challenges may arise in June, but taking time for yourself will help. Later in the month, opportunities will present themselves, so be ready to act on them. Be cautious with financial matters.

SNAKE

Positive energy is vital in June, enhancing creativity and luck. Financial energy improves, though caution is still advised with risks. Relationships will thrive, and confidence will be critical to your success.

HORSE

This month, networking is emphasised, and job changes are favoured. Recognition and essential connections are likely. Take time to rest later in the month to recover from accumulated fatigue.

9
Monday

Animal: **Earth Rooster**
Flying Star: **4**
Good Day: **Dragon**
Bad Day: **Rabbit**
💇🖤❤️

10
Tuesday

Animal: **Metal Dog**
Flying Star: **5**
Good Day: **Rabbit**
Bad Day: **Dragon**
⚡💰🏠✂️✈️🎬

11
Wednesday

Animal: **Metal Pig**
Flying Star: **6**
Good Day: **Tiger**
Bad Day: **Snake**
🏠✈️🎬

12
Thursday

Animal: **Water Rat**
Flying Star: **7**
Good Day: **Ox**
Bad Day: **Horse**

13
Friday

Animal: **Water Ox**
Flying Star: **8**
Good Day: **Rat**
Bad Day: **Goat**
✂️🎉🎬

14
Saturday

Animal: **Wood Tiger**
Flying Star: **9**
Good Day: **Pig**
Bad Day: **Monkey**
✂️🎉🎬

15
Sunday

Animal: **Wood Rabbit**
Flying Star: **1**
Good Day: **Dog**
Bad Day: **Rooster**

GOAT

June brings more supportive energy than previous months. Financial gains are possible, but caution is still necessary. Focus on strengthening your position and managing resources wisely.

MONKEY

June may be turbulent, requiring a gentle and sincere approach to succeed. Relationships can be stressful, so manage emotions carefully. Take time to relax and care for your well-being.

ROOSTER

June starts slowly, but an energy shift is on the horizon. Focus on social interactions and new connections could lead to valuable opportunities. Maintain work-life balance for optimal results.

DOG

June marks a favourable period of busy work and social activities. A positive mindset will help you maximise the month's opportunities. Personal relationships will flourish.

PIG

June's supportive energy will boost your confidence. Your financial prospects are moderate but stable. Enjoy the outdoors, but prioritise personal safety, especially in risky activities.

06 | JUNE 2025

The Wood Snake Year

16
Monday

Animal: **Fire Dragon**
Flying Star: **2**
Good Day: **Rooster**
Bad Day: **Dog**

17
Tuesday

Animal: **Fire Snake**
Flying Star: **3**
Good Day: **Monkey**
Bad Day: **Pig**
🏯

18
Wednesday

Animal: **Earth Horse**
Flying Star: **4**
Good Day: **Goat**
Bad Day: **Rat**
🐖❤️

19
Thursday

Animal: **Earth Goat**
Flying Star: **5**
Good Day: **Horse**
Bad Day: **Ox**
⚡✈️🏠🥏✒️🎉

20
Friday

Animal: **Metal Monkey**
Flying Star: **6**
Good Day: **Snake**
Bad Day: **Tiger**
✈️🏠🥏🎉

21
Saturday

Animal: **Metal Rooster**
Flying Star: **0**
Good Day: **Dragon**
Bad Day: **Rabbit**
🐿️🥏

22
Sunday

Animal: **Water Dog**
Flying Star: **2**
Good Day: **Rabbit**
Bad Day: **Dragon**
✈️🏠🥢🥏✒️

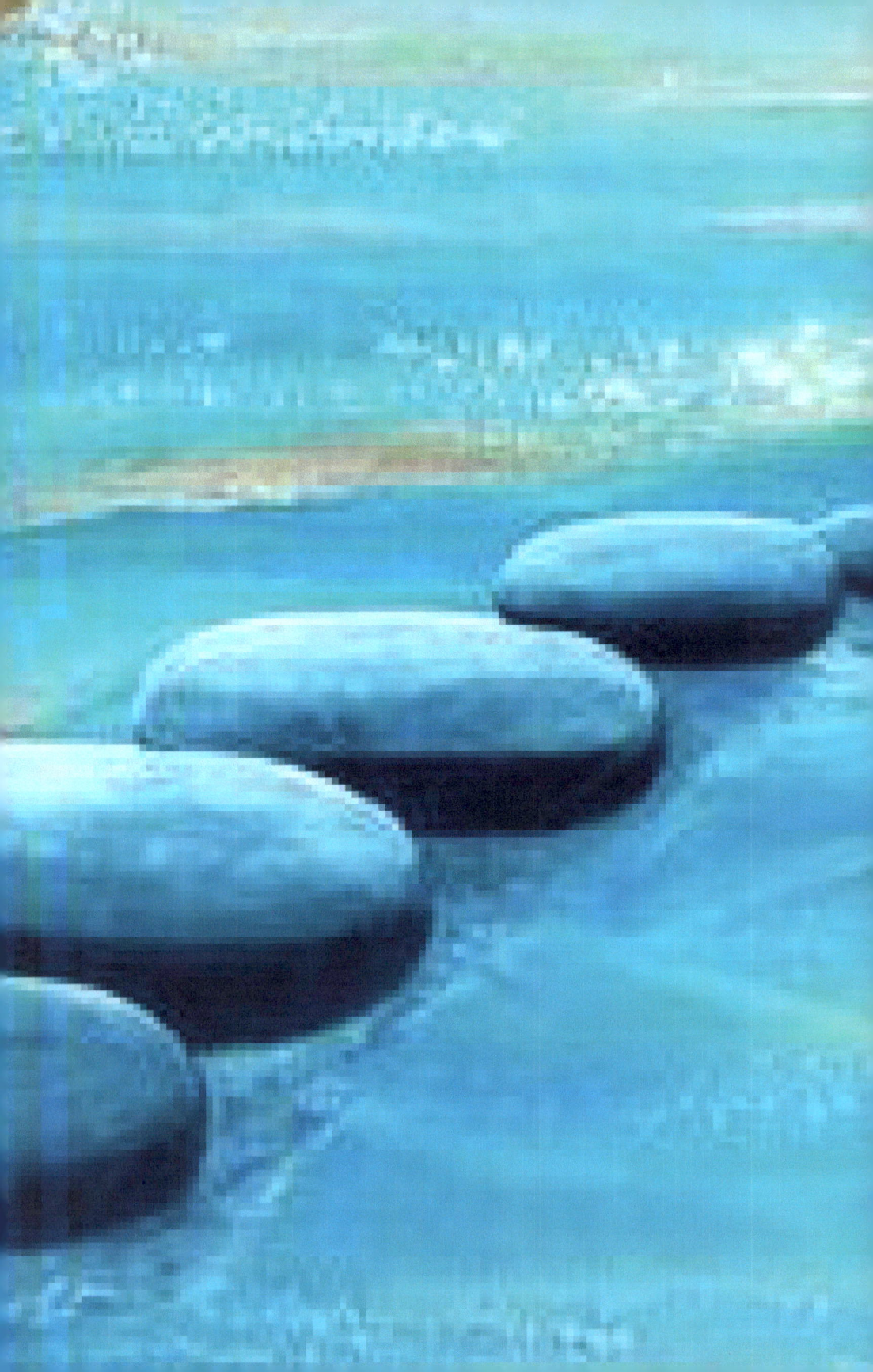

The Wood Snake Year

23
Monday

Animal: **Water Pig**
Flying Star: **1**
Good Day: **Tiger**
Bad Day: **Snake**

24
Tuesday

Animal: **Wood Rat**
Flying Star: **9**
Good Day: **Ox**
Bad Day: **Horse**

25
Wednesday

Animal: **Wood Ox**
Flying Star: **8**
Good Day: **Rat**
Bad Day: **Goat**

26
Thursday

Animal: **Fire Tiger**
Flying Star: **7**
Good Day: **Pig**
Bad Day: **Monkey**

27
Friday

Animal: **Fire Rabbit**
Flying Star: **6**
Good Day: **Dog**
Bad Day: **Rooster**

28
Saturday

Animal: **Earth Dragon**
Flying Star: **5**
Good Day: **Rooster**
Bad Day: **Dog**

29
Sunday

Animal: **Earth Snake**
Flying Star: **4**
Good Day: **Monkey**
Bad Day: **Pig**

July 7 - August 7 is the Month of the Goat

Goat Chinese Horoscope 2025: Flourishing with the Fire Snake

Goat Birth Years: 1919, 1931, 1943, 1955, 1967, 1979, 1991, 2003, 2015, 2027, 2039

In 2025, the Goat will experience the vibrant and transformative energy of the Yin Wood-Snake. This year shifts from the stable influences of the Wood Dragon in 2024, bringing a dynamic and passionate atmosphere that will affect various aspects of life for the Goat.

Fire Snake Influence: Passion and Creativity

The Year of the Yin Wood Snake introduces a period of intense transformation and creativity for the Goat. The Fire Snake's fiery and enigmatic energy contrasts with the more steady Dragon of 2024, encouraging the Goats to embrace passion and innovation in their pursuits.

Career and Opportunities: Embracing Innovation

For Goats, 2025 offers exciting career opportunities fuelled by the Fire Snake's influence. The year favours bold decisions and creative approaches. Goats should leverage their natural adaptability and determination to embrace new projects and ideas. The Fire Snake's energy allows one to explore innovative career paths and achieve significant growth.

Wealth and Prosperity: Strategic Growth

Financially, the Year of the Fire Snake presents a mixed landscape. While growth opportunities are available, the Fire Snake's unpredictable nature calls for strategic planning and caution. Goats should avoid risky investments and focus on stable and well-researched financial strategies. Patience and careful management will be essential for achieving financial success.

Love and Relationships: Intensity and Connection

The Fire Snake's passionate energy brings a dynamic shift in love and relationships. For single Goats, this year offers the possibility of intense and transformative connections. Building trust and open communication will be crucial. For those in committed relationships, the Fire Snake's influence may lead to emotional intensity, requiring patience and understanding to navigate potential challenges.

Social Dynamics and Harmony: Building Connections

The Fire Snake's influence enhances the Goat's social interactions, encouraging deeper connections and meaningful relationships. Goats should embrace their natural kindness and adaptability to strengthen bonds with friends and family. This year is ideal for expanding social networks and participating in community activities.

Health and Well-being: Balancing Energy

Maintaining health and well-being will be crucial with the Fire Snake's intense energy. Goats should balance their physical and emotional health through exercise, stress management, and a healthy diet. Paying attention to self-care and adapting to the year's energetic shifts will support overall vitality.

Symbolism of the Goat and Fire Snake: Transformation and Growth

In 2025, the Goat's endurance and adaptability blend with the Fire Snake's passion and creativity. This year symbolises a period of profound transformation and opportunity. Goats can achieve significant personal and professional growth by harnessing the Fire Snake's dynamic energy and embracing change.

2025: A Year of Passion and Transformation

The Year of the Yin Wood Snake offers the Goat a vibrant and transformative experience. Embracing innovation, maintaining strategic financial planning, and nurturing relationships will be vital to thriving in this energetic year. With the Fire Snake's influence, Goats are poised for a year of exciting growth and opportunity.

JULY, Flying Star 6: A Radiant Beacon of Authority and Fortune

July ushers in the illustrious Flying Star 6, a celestial force that brings the energies of authority, power, wealth, and heavenly luck. This star is a harbinger of prosperous times, orchestrating a grand symphony of career opportunities and the realisation of long-held ambitions. Under its glowing influence, one can expect an infusion of enhanced power, elevated status, and the radiant aura of a commendable reputation. As an emissary of prosperity, Flying Star 6 bestows divine favour upon its beneficiaries, particularly those seeking career advancement and success. Middle-aged women, middle daughters, and those born under the Horse zodiac sign are especially poised to reap the rewards of this star's benevolent influence.

The veneration of Flying Star 6's positive attributes can establish a commanding presence, symbolising elevated status and influential sway within professional and social circles. Its energetic current encapsulates the essence of authority, empowering individuals to step into leadership roles and distinction.

To fully awaken the potential of Flying Star 6, one must infuse it with vibrant Yang energy. This can be achieved through the harmonious interplay of water features, resonant sounds, and lively activities. Traditional enhancers, steeped in symbolism, can amplify this star's auspicious energies—whether through the dignified presence of a Horse figurine, the subtle charm of Six Gold Coins suspended from a tassel, or the enduring symbol of Gold Ingots.

However, despite its brilliance, caution is advised. External negative influences can unexpectedly cast shadows over Flying Star 6, turning its blessings into turbulent challenges. Such disruptions may manifest as sudden upheavals, abrupt changes, or even medical complications related to the kidneys or legs.

As Flying Star 6 radiates its potent energies in July, embracing its power with wisdom and awareness can lead to prosperity, authority, and enduring success.

In 2025, the annual Flying Star 6 will grace the South sector of the Luo Shu or Bagua School of Feng Shui, a domain traditionally associated with fame, recognition, and reputation. The Fire element governs this sector and is symbolically represented by the celestial red phoenix.

Enhancing your home's southern area to harness this sector's potent energies is advantageous. This can be achieved by strategically using the Phoenix statue or imagery of horses, which embody the speed and endurance essential for success. Embracing bright lighting and incorporating red or fire-coloured objects will amplify the sector's influence. Additionally, integrating wood elements like plants will harmonise the interaction between water and fire energies, fostering a balanced environment. Including galloping horse symbols is particularly effective, as it invigorates your pursuits and motivates you to achieve recognition and acclaim throughout 2025.

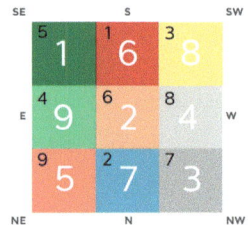

SE	S	SW
5 / **1**	1 / **6**	3 / **8**
4 / **9** (E)	6 / **2**	8 / **4** (W)
9 / **5** (NE)	2 / **7** (N)	7 / **3** (NW)

30 Monday

Animal: **Metal Horse**
Flying Star: **3**
Good Day: **Goat**
Bad Day: **Rat**
✈️

1 Tuesday

Animal: **Metal Goat**
Flying Star: **2**
Good Day: **Horse**
Bad Day: **Ox**
✈️🏠🪙✂️🛏️🎬

2 Wednesday

Animal: **Water Monkey**
Flying Star: **1**
Good Day: **Snake**
Bad Day: **Tiger**
🎉

3 Thursday

Animal: **Water Rooster**
Flying Star: **9**
Good Day: **Dragon**
Bad Day: **Rabbit**
💇

4 Friday

Animal: **Wood Dog**
Flying Star: **8**
Good Day: **Rabbit**
Bad Day: **Dragon**
✈️🏠✂️🪙🎬

5 Saturday

Animal: **Wood Pig**
Flying Star: **7**
Good Day: **Tiger**
Bad Day: **Snake**
✈️🏠🎬

6 Sunday

Animal: **Fire Rat**
Flying Star: **6**
Good Day: **Ox**
Bad Day: **Horse**

JULY MONTHLY CHINESE ZODIAC OVERVIEW

RAT

The fast-paced energy of July may cloud your thinking, so it's crucial to stay patient and thorough, especially with financial matters. Leaders managing large teams may need extra support. To maintain personal well-being, consider a short vacation or recharge in nature.

OX

July brings mixed energy—strong support and success in some areas but sudden challenges in others. Be aware of tough competition at work, and avoid risky projects. Consider taking time off to recharge and maintain your focus for a productive month.

TIGER

July's energy is intense but emotionally draining. Pacing yourself will help you achieve goals more efficiently. Work issues from the past will start to settle, and if you feel sluggish, a few days off could provide a much-needed refresh.

RABBIT

This month brings luck and support from those around you. New opportunities are likely, and you'll need to act decisively to advance. Financial energy is favourable, with possible windfall gains or successful investments.

DRAGON

July will improve your life significantly. Work and business will see growth, supported by wealth and energy. In your personal life, focus on avoiding conflicts with loved ones or friends to keep harmony intact.

SNAKE

July brings unstable energy that may increase stress at work. It's essential to manage stress effectively and avoid overworking. Personal relationships may face challenges, so ensure open communication and self-care to prevent emotional strain.

HORSE

This month's energy is mixed and may lead to confusion. Stay calm and adapt to changing circumstances. Travelling to visit friends or family can offer a fresh perspective and help you manage the month's fluctuations.

The Wood Snake Year

7
Monday

Animal: **Fire Ox**
Flying Star: **5**
Good Day: **Rat**
Bad Day: **Goat**
⚡

8
Tuesday

Animal: **Earth Tiger**
Flying Star: **4**
Good Day: **Pig**
Bad Day: **Monkey**
✈️ 💅 🏠 👙 ❤️ 💍 ✂️ 🎉 🎬

9
Wednesday

Animal: **Earth Rabbit**
Flying Star: **3**
Good Day: **Dog**
Bad Day: **Rooster**
🏠 ✈️ 💍 ✂️ 🎉 🎬

10
Thursday

Animal: **Metal Dragon**
Flying Star: **2**
Good Day: **Rooster**
Bad Day: **Dog**

11
Friday

Animal: **Metal Snake**
Flying Star: **1**
Good Day: **Monkey**
Bad Day: **Pig**
💅 🎉

12
Saturday

Animal: **Water Horse**
Flying Star: **9**
Good Day: **Goat**
Bad Day: **Rat**
🎬

13
Sunday

Animal: **Water Goat**
Flying Star: **8**
Good Day: **Horse**
Bad Day: **Ox**
✈️ 💍

GOAT

July is a lucky and productive month for you. Embrace this time with creativity and infuse joy into everything you do. On a personal level, a new chapter may be beginning, requiring life adjustments for the better.

MONKEY

July brings exciting energy and the opportunity to see the fruits of your past efforts. Use this time for personal growth and advancement. Wealth energy is stable, and you'll have a solid foundation for future success.

ROOSTER

Unstable energy in July may cause worry and sleeplessness. To regain balance, focus on self-care and regulate your activities. Avoid making major changes at work and be cautious with large expenditures or investments.

DOG

Work may present challenges this month, but persistence will bring progress. Spend time decluttering your home or workspace to shift stagnant energy. Keep a positive attitude, as growth opportunities will emerge by staying focused.

PIG

July's energy brings a positive outlook. Exciting events and social activities will keep you busy, while work projects will progress smoothly. Enjoy this lighter, favourable period, boosting your overall health and happiness.

14
Monday

Animal: **Wood Monkey**
Flying Star: **7**
Good Day: **Snake**
Bad Day: **Tiger**
🏠🐎🧧🎆🎬

15
Tuesday

Animal: **Wood Rooster**
Flying Star: **6**
Good Day: **Dragon**
Bad Day: **Rabbit**
💇🧧🎉

16
Wednesday

Animal: **Fire Dog**
Flying Star: **5**
Good Day: **Rabbit**
Bad Day: **Dragon**
⚡

17
Thursday

Animal: **Fire Pig**
Flying Star: **4**
Good Day: **Tiger**
Bad Day: **Snake**
🎬🦇❤️

18
Friday

Animal: **Earth Rat**
Flying Star: **3**
Good Day: **Ox**
Bad Day: **Horse**
🎬💇

19
Saturday

Animal: **Earth Ox**
Flying Star: **2**
Good Day: **Rat**
Bad Day: **Goat**

20
Sunday

Animal: **Metal Tiger**
Flying Star: **1**
Good Day: **Pig**
Bad Day: **Monkey**
✈️🧧🎆🎬

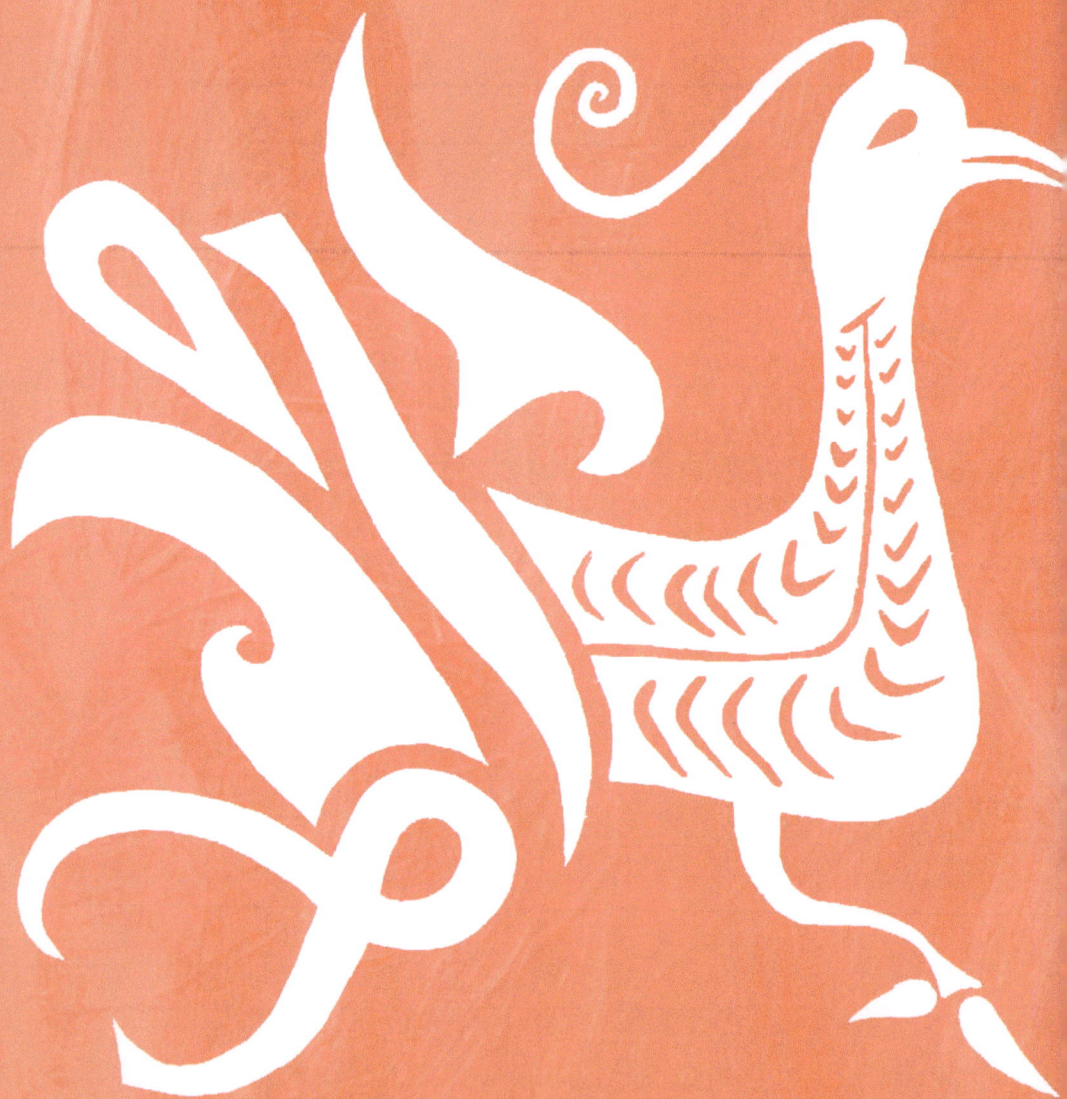

21
Monday

Animal: **Metal Rabbit**
Flying Star: **9**
Good Day: **Dog**
Bad Day: **Dragon**
✈️🏠🕶️🚗✂️🎆🎬

22
Tuesday

Animal: **Water Dragon**
Flying Star: **8**
Good Day: **Rooster**
Bad Day: **Dog**
🚗

23
Wednesday

Animal: **Water Snake**
Flying Star: **7**
Good Day: **Monkey**
Bad Day: **Pig**
🕶️🎬

24
Thursday

Animal: **Wood Horse**
Flying Star: **6**
Good Day: **Goat**
Bad Day: **Rat**

25
Friday

Animal: **Wood Goat**
Flying Star: **5**
Good Day: **Horse**
Bad Day: **Ox**
⚡✈️🕶️🚗

26
Saturday

Animal: **Fire Monkey**
Flying Star: **4**
Good Day: **Snake**
Bad Day: **Tiger**
🎬🪷❤️🚗

27
Sunday

Animal: **Fire Rooster**
Flying Star: **3**
Good Day: **Dragon**
Bad Day: **Rabbit**
✈️🚗✂️🕶️🎆

August 8 – September 7 is the Month of the Monkey

Monkey Chinese Horoscope 2025: Embracing Transformation and Passion

Monkey Birth Years: 1920, 1932, 1944, 1956, 1968, 1980, 1992, 2004, 2016, 2028, 2040

In 2025, the Monkey will navigate the energetic and transformative influence of the Yin Wood-Snake. This year marks a departure from the grounded and stable Wood Dragon of 2024, introducing a vibrant and intense atmosphere that will shape the Monkey's experiences.

Fire Snake Influence: Transformation and Passion

The Year of the Yin Wood Snake infuses the Monkey's life with dynamic energy and creative possibilities. The Fire Snake's passionate and transformative nature encourages Monkeys to embrace change and innovation. This is a year for exploring new ideas and pursuing goals with enthusiasm.

Career Focus: Innovation and Strategic Moves

For Monkeys, the Year of the Fire Snake presents significant career opportunities driven by creativity and strategic thinking. This is a prime time for Monkeys to harness their ingenuity and adaptability to advance professionally. Embracing new challenges, networking with influential figures, and pursuing innovative projects will be crucial to career success.

Love and Relationships: Intense Connections

In love, the Fire Snake's influence brings intensity and transformation. Single Monkeys may experience exciting romantic prospects characterised by passionate and transformative connections. Those in committed relationships should be prepared for emotional depth and potential challenges. Open communication, patience, and understanding will be crucial for nurturing relationships.

Finance Strategies: Caution and Opportunity

Financially, the Year of the Fire Snake presents both opportunities and risks. While there are potential avenues for financial growth, Monkeys should approach investments cautiously. Strategic planning and careful research are essential to avoid unnecessary risks. Balancing bold financial moves with prudent management will be necessary for maintaining economic stability.

Health and Well-being: Balancing Energy

With the Fire Snake's intense energy, maintaining health and well-being requires attention to balance. Monkeys should focus on managing stress, maintaining a healthy lifestyle, and incorporating regular exercise into their routines. Adequate rest and self-care will support overall vitality and help navigate the energetic shifts of the year.

Symbolism of the Monkey and Fire Snake: Transformation and Innovation

In 2025, the Monkey's adaptability and resourcefulness blend with the Fire Snake's passionate and transformative energy. This year symbolises a time of significant change and creative growth. By embracing innovation and navigating challenges with enthusiasm, Monkeys can make the most of the opportunities presented by the Fire Snake.

2025: A Year of Passion and Transformation

The Year of the Yin Wood Snake offers the Monkey a vibrant and transformative experience. Embracing change, pursuing creative ventures, and managing finances cautiously will be vital to thriving in this dynamic year. With the Fire Snake's influence, Monkeys are poised for a year of exciting growth and opportunities.

AUGUST, Flying Star 5: A Star of Dark Omens and Harbingers of Misfortune

In August, the menacing energy of Flying Star 5 reclaims the spotlight, weaving its way into the intricate tapestry of cosmic influences. Known as the infamous 5 Yellow Star, this celestial force casts a foreboding shadow over all it touches. It is one of the most treacherous and aggressive stars in Feng Shui, renowned for ushering in danger, misfortune, and disruptive forces. The reputation of Flying Star 5 precedes it—a harbinger of woes, a bringer of bad luck, and a weaver of calamities.

As this ominous star unfurls its dark energy, it sets the stage for adversity and hindrances, spreading its evil influence across all aspects of life. Its toxic aura attracts unfavourable outcomes, with the youngest son and those born under the Ox and Tiger zodiac signs particularly vulnerable to its pernicious effects. The misfortunes it brings are vast and disheartening, ranging from financial loss and business disruptions to betrayals, tragic accidents, and even fatal calamities.

A palpable sense of dread surrounds Flying Star 5, as it embodies an array of negative energies that can envelop one's endeavours in a shroud of despair. This star symbolises bankruptcy, disloyalty, and other harbingers of doom that threaten to topple even the most stable foundations.

Ancient Feng Shui wisdom offers valuable guidance to guard against its ominous influence. Breaking ground or initiating new renovation projects under this star's presence is strongly discouraged, as it may unleash its potent negativity. The most effective strategy is to let this star lie dormant and undisturbed, minimising interaction with its energy. However, when avoidance isn't possible, remedies can be employed to mitigate its effects. The Brass Pagoda, the solemn tones of a bronze bell, the harmonious melody of metal wind chimes, and the purifying Saltwater Cure all serve as potent countermeasures. Additionally, invoking the benevolent presence of Ganesha, the remover of obstacles, can provide solace and protection.

To further counteract the grip of this adversarial star, heavy metal objects made of brass, copper, bronze, or pewter can be strategically placed in the Northeast sector of the home. Incorporating metallic artwork, decor, and colours that resonate with resistance can help diminish its influence. Simultaneously, minimising Fire and Earth energies in this area will weaken its potency, ensuring a safer and more harmonious environment during the star's reign.

For 2025, the Northeast sector of the Luo Shu or Bagua School of Feng Shui holds great significance as it hosts the annual Flying Star 5, a symbol of knowledge, scholarly pursuits, learning, and education. This presents a prime opportunity for Feng Shui adjustments that could usher in positive transformations in these areas, instilling homeowners a renewed sense of hope and optimism.

The Northeast, governed by the Earth element, may become unstable with excessive Earth energy. However, a proactive approach can restore balance and harness its potential. To fortify this sector, consider incorporating imagery of mountains, a crystal globe, a world map, the Chinese saint Luohan, or Dragon Carp. These elements can enhance and support the area's energy. Additionally, be mindful of any large trees or missing spaces that might obstruct this sector, as addressing these issues will be crucial in tapping into its full potential. Your deliberate efforts can significantly influence your home's energy and its impact on your life.

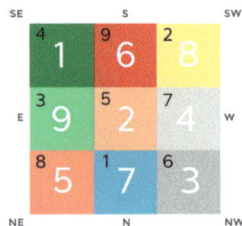

28
Monday

Animal: **Earth Dog**
Flying Star: **2**
Good Day: **Rabbit**
Bad Day: **Dragon**

29
Tuesday

Animal: **Earth Pig**
Flying Star: **1**
Good Day: **Tiger**
Bad Day: **Snake**

30
Wednesday

Animal: **Metal Rat**
Flying Star: **9**
Good Day: **Ox**
Bad Day: **Horse**

31
Thursday

Animal: **Metal Ox**
Flying Star: **8**
Good Day: **Rat**
Bad Day: **Goat**

1
Friday

Animal: **Water Tiger**
Flying Star: **7**
Good Day: **Pig**
Bad Day: **Monkey**

2
Saturday

Animal: **Water Rabbit**
Flying Star: **6**
Good Day: **Dog**
Bad Day: **Rooster**

3
Sunday

Animal: **Wood Dragon**
Flying Star: **5**
Good Day: **Rooster**
Bad Day: **Dog**

AUGUST MONTHLY CHINESE ZODIAC OVERVIEW

RAT

As energy speeds up in August, stay mindful of personal safety. Be aware of potential challenges in your interactions and handle them with gentleness. Avoid hasty decisions or actions, as this month requires a calm and steady approach.

OX

August starts with some instability, but your situation will improve as the month progresses. Your career and business will see positive growth, but manage your finances carefully. Avoid high-risk activities to protect your safety.

TIGER

The energy this month may drain you emotionally, affecting your sleep patterns. Work or business could slow down, and financial concerns might arise. To reduce stress, avoid crowded or overly stimulating environments.

RABBIT

August brings challenges that will test your vision and encourage change. If you've been considering a career shift, now is an excellent time to pursue it. Partnerships and joint ventures will thrive, offering success in collaboration.

DRAGON

Fluctuating energy this month may cause some uneasiness. Stay strong and positive to prevent chaos from creeping in. Take a step back to allow personal energy to settle, and you'll soon see the positive aspects emerging. Prioritise safety and security during this time.

SNAKE

Opportunities will present themselves this month, but you must remain alert. Be mindful of personal safety as you navigate busy schedules. Travel is on the horizon, so avoid accidents during journeys.

HORSE

You may feel a surge of creative energy, leading to new projects and innovative ideas. Embrace this inspiration and use it to maximise your professional endeavours. Financial energy is favourable, so there's potential for increased earnings or successful investments.

The Wood Snake Year

4
Monday

Animal: **Wood Snake**
Flying Star: **4**
Good Day: **Monkey**
Bad Day: **Pig**
💍❤️🩲

5
Tuesday

Animal: **Fire Horse**
Flying Star: **3**
Good Day: **Goat**
Bad Day: **Rat**
🎬

6
Wednesday

Animal: **Fire Goat**
Flying Star: **2**
Good Day: **Horse**
Bad Day: **Ox**
✈️

7
Thursday

Animal: **Earth Monkey**
Flying Star: **1**
Good Day: **Snake**
Bad Day: **Tiger**
✈️🏠

8
Friday

Animal: **Earth Rooster**
Flying Star: **9**
Good Day: **Dragon**
Bad Day: **Rabbit**
🐿️🎬

9
Saturday

Animal: **Metal Dog**
Flying Star: **8**
Good Day: **Rabbit**
Bad Day: **Dragon**

10
Sunday

Animal: **Metal Pig**
Flying Star: **7**
Good Day: **Tiger**
Bad Day: **Snake**

GOAT

Instability this month may unsettle you, especially regarding finances. It's a good time to budget carefully and avoid significant investments. Focus on planning and preparation to maintain financial stability throughout the month.

MONKEY

Although some changes may affect your projects, August brings a wave of optimism. Approach these transitions calmly and maintain clear communication with those involved. Relationships will experience harmony and growth.

ROOSTER

August's energy is favourable, bringing rapid progress and success in business and social activities. Be mindful of your thoughts—positive energy will attract more positivity. Aim to elevate your personal and professional standards for long-term success.

DOG

August's mixed energy will require careful management. Stay active and enthusiastic to balance fluctuations. New people or relationships may enter your life, but financial energy remains weak, so manage your resources carefully.

PIG

This month's energy can be challenging to control, so moderate your expectations. Opportunities may arise, but money energy is low, so avoid major financial decisions. Prioritise your health, especially if you have pre-existing conditions.

11
Monday

Animal: **Water Rat**
Flying Star: **6**
Good Day: **Ox**
Bad Day: **Horse**
✈️🏭

12
Tuesday

Animal: **Water Ox**
Flying Star: **5**
Good Day: **Rat**
Bad Day: **Goat**
🏭⚡

13
Wednesday

Animal: **Wood Tiger**
Flying Star: **4**
Good Day: **Pig**
Bad Day: **Monkey**
❤️🐀

14
Thursday

Animal: **Wood Rabbit**
Flying Star: **3**
Good Day: **Dog**
Bad Day: **Rooster**

15
Friday

Animal: **Fire Dragon**
Flying Star: **2**
Good Day: **Rooster**
Bad Day: **Dog**
🏠🎉🥢🚗/🏭

16
Saturday

Animal: **Fire Snake**
Flying Star: **1**
Good Day: **Monkey**
Bad Day: **Pig**
🏠🥢/🎉

17
Sunday

Animal: **Fire Horse**
Flying Star: **9**
Good Day: **Goat**
Bad Day: **Rat**
✈️🥢

IDEAL KITCHEN PLACEMENT IN FENG SHUI

In feng shui, the kitchen is often considered an inauspicious area due to potentially harmful energy generated during activities such as cutting vegetables and meat, washing, and accumulating garbage before disposal. Despite this, kitchens play a crucial role, as strategically placing them in less auspicious locations can help mitigate any potential negative influences in those sectors.

It is essential to avoid placing the kitchen in sectors where it might obstruct access to positive energy. When buying a new home or undertaking renovations, it is advisable to position the kitchen in less favourable areas of the home.

IMPORTANT: Kitchens should never be located in the Northwest (NW) sector, as it signifies 'Fire At Heaven's Gate,' which can harm the Patriarch. Adhering to this principle is a fundamental rule in feng shui.

Optimal Kitchen Locations Based on House-Facing Direction:

North:	SW, W, NE
Northeast:	E, SE, S, N
East:	NE, W, SW
Southeast:	W, NE, SW
South:	SW, NE, W
Southwest:	S, N, E, SE
West:	SE, E, N, S
Northwest:	N, S, SW, E

Kitchen placement should align with the house-facing direction. Remember, the one rule that must not be broken is never locating the kitchen in the NW sector.

18
Monday

Animal: **Earth Goat**
Flying Star: **8**
Good Day: **Horse**
Bad Day: **Ox**
🏬

19
Tuesday

Animal: **Earth Monkey**
Flying Star: **7**
Good Day: **Snake**
Bad Day: **Tiger**
✈️

20
Wednesday

Animal: **Metal Rooster**
Flying Star: **6**
Good Day: **Dragon**
Bad Day: **Rabbit**
🏬

21
Thursday

Animal: **Metal Dog**
Flying Star: **5**
Good Day: **Rabbit**
Bad Day: **Dragon**
⚡✈️🏠

22
Friday

Animal: **Water Pig**
Flying Star: **4**
Good Day: **Tiger**
Bad Day: **Snake**
❤️🤝

23
Saturday

Animal: **Water Rat**
Flying Star: **3**
Good Day: **Ox**
Bad Day: **Horse**
✈️🏠🤝✂️🏬

24
Sunday

Animal: **Wood Ox**
Flying Star: **2**
Good Day: **Rat**
Bad Day: **Goat**
🏬

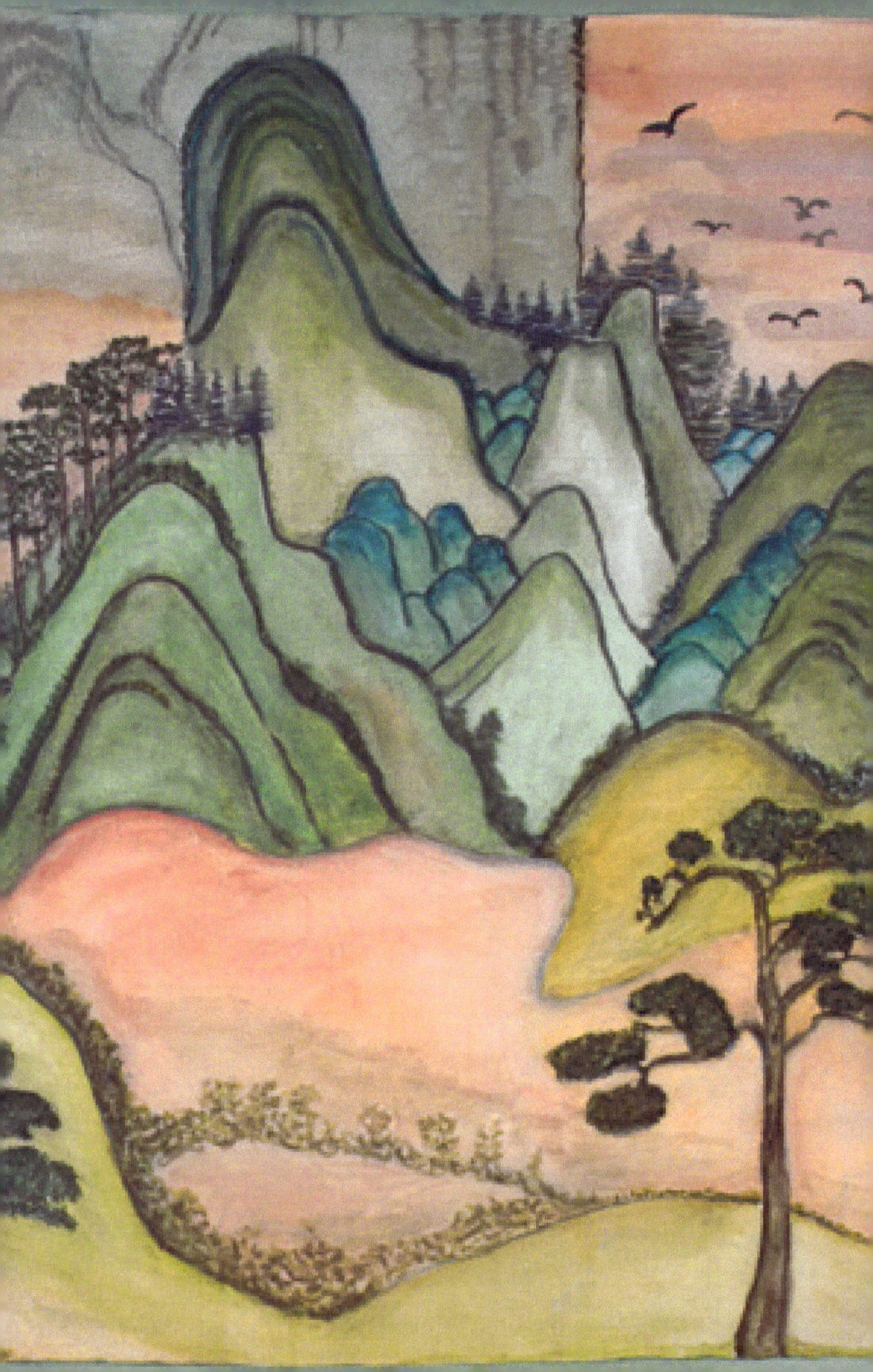

08 | AUGUST
2025

The Wood Snake Year

25
Monday

Animal: **Wood Tiger**
Flying Star: **1**
Good Day: **Pig**
Bad Day: **Monkey**

26
Tuesday

Animal: **Fire Rabbit**
Flying Star: **9**
Good Day: **Dog**
Bad Day: **Rooster**
✈🏠🐚➰✂🎉

27
Wednesday

Animal: **Fire Dragon**
Flying Star: **8**
Good Day: **Rooster**
Bad Day: **Dog**
✈🏠➰✂🎉🏰

28
Thursday

Animal: **Earth Snake**
Flying Star: **7**
Good Day: **Monkey**
Bad Day: **Pig**
🏠🐚➰✂🏰

29
Friday

Animal: **Earth Horse**
Flying Star: **6**
Good Day: **Goat**
Bad Day: **Rat**
✈🐕🐚🏰

30
Saturday

Animal: **Metal Goat**
Flying Star: **5**
Good Day: **Horse**
Bad Day: **Ox**
⚡✈🏰

31
Sunday

Animal: **Metal Monkey**
Flying Star: **4**
Good Day: **Snake**
Bad Day: **Tiger**
✈🏠❤🩲🐚

September 8 – October 7 is the Month of the Rooster

Rooster Chinese Horoscope 2025: Embracing Passion and Transformation

Rooster Birth Years: 1921, 1933, 1945, 1957, 1969, 1981, 1993, 2005, 2017, 2029, 2041

In 2025, the Rooster will experience the energetic and transformative influences of the Yin Wood-Snake. This year brings a shift from the grounded and stable Dragon of 2024 to a more dynamic and passionate environment, offering opportunities and challenges.

Fire Snake Influence: Passion and Innovation

The Year of the Yin Wood Snake introduces an atmosphere of intensity and transformation. The Fire Snake's influence encourages the Rooster to embrace creativity and innovation, pushing them to explore new paths and make bold decisions. This year is about harnessing passionate energy for personal and professional growth.

Career Focus: Creativity and Adaptability

For Roosters, the Year of the Fire Snake highlights the importance of creativity and adaptability in their careers. This is a time to leverage new ideas, pursue innovative projects, and take calculated risks. Networking and forming strategic alliances will be beneficial. While opportunities for advancement are present, Roosters should remain adaptable to navigate the dynamic professional landscape effectively.

Love and Relationships: Intense and Transformative

The Fire Snake brings intense and transformative energy to matters of love. Single Roosters may encounter passionate and potentially life-changing romantic prospects. Existing relationships may undergo significant changes, requiring open communication and emotional depth. Roosters should focus on building strong connections and addressing any underlying issues for a harmonious year in love.

Finance Strategies: Caution and Opportunity

Financially, the Year of the Fire Snake presents potential gains and risks. Roosters should exercise caution in financial decisions, avoiding impulsive investments and focusing on strategic planning. Innovative approaches and careful research can lead to profitable opportunities. Maintaining a balanced budget and avoiding unnecessary expenditures will be crucial for financial stability.

Health and Well-being: Balancing Passion and Care

With the Fire Snake's intense energy, maintaining health and well-being requires focusing on balance. Roosters should manage stress, incorporate regular exercise, and prioritise self-care. Finding time for relaxation and ensuring a nutritious diet will support overall health. Engaging in mental and emotional respite activities will help maintain well-being throughout the year.

Symbolism of the Rooster and Fire Snake: Passion and Transformation

The Rooster's energetic and diligent nature combines the Fire Snake's transformative and passionate influence in 2025. This year symbolises a period of significant change and creative growth. By embracing the Fire Snake's energy, Roosters can make substantial strides in their personal and professional lives.

2025: A Year of Dynamic Growth

The Year of the Yin Wood Snake offers Roosters a year filled with dynamic energy and transformative opportunities. Embracing innovation, navigating challenges with adaptability, and maintaining a balanced approach to finances and health will help Roosters make the most of the vibrant and intense atmosphere of 2025.

SEPTEMBER, Flying Star 4: A Symphony of Romance, Wisdom, and Scholarly Flourish

In September, the celestial energies align to bring forth the harmonious influence of Flying Star 4, a beacon of romance, wisdom, and intellectual brilliance. Emerging as a graceful melody within the cosmic symphony, this star weaves an intricate tapestry of love, intelligence, talent, and scholarly achievement. Known as the Peach Blossom Star, Flying Star 4 radiates beauty and knowledge, enriching the lives of those it touches and infusing the environment with grace and charm.

As the energies of Flying Star 4 permeate your surroundings, love and relationships take on an enchanting glow. Its benevolent presence nurtures meaningful connections, fostering harmony and happiness in romantic endeavours. This star promises love blossoming and deepening emotional bonds, which is exceptionally favourable for those born under the Rooster sign and the youngest daughter. For singles, it offers the prospect of finding a soulmate, while couples find their connection strengthened under its gentle influence.

Beyond the realm of the heart, Flying Star 4 extends its blessings to those with artistic, literary, or intellectual pursuits. Educators, artists, writers, and researchers are poised to benefit from its favourable energies, opening doors to advancement, recognition, and new opportunities. Students, too, find themselves under its supportive wing, enjoying enhanced luck in exams and tremendous success in academic endeavours. The star's touch enhances creativity and intellect, making it a powerful ally for those seeking wisdom and scholarly achievement.

To amplify this star's romantic energy, couples are encouraged to adorn their spaces with symbols of love. Placing two Rose Quartz crystals near the bed invokes the power of affection and harmony. At the same time, love symbols such as Mandarin Ducks, Wish-fulfilling Birds, or embracing figurines remind us of the tender connection between partners.

For those seeking academic success, Flying Star 4 offers a guiding light. Displaying Chinese ink brushes, artistic creations, tiered pagodas, or symbols of revered figures like the Chinese saint Luohan or the three Star Gods can help harmonise with the star's essence. These tokens act as conduits, channelling the star's energy to illuminate the path to academic excellence and intellectual growth.

In September, Flying Star 4 invites you to embrace its gifts of love, wisdom, and creativity, transforming your environment into a sanctuary of romance and scholarly brilliance.

In 2025, the Western sector of the Luo Shu or Bagua School of Feng Shui will emerge significantly. This sector, graced by the annual Flying Star 4, embodies the themes of family, descendants, and safeguarding wealth and assets. This insight allows for strategic Feng Shui adjustments, providing you with the foresight to prepare and enhance your environment for the year ahead.

The Western sector is the domain of the celestial white Tiger, making it vital to incorporate Tiger symbolism here to fortify and protect family luck. In this area, place wealth-related symbols such as Gold Coins, Gold Ingots, or a Wealth God to bolster wealth and ensure the family's well-being. The Western sector is associated with the Metal element, so integrating metallic artwork, paintings, or colours, as well as displaying family photos in metallic frames, will harmonise and enhance the energy of this space.

SE	S	SW
3 **1**	8 **6**	1 **8**
2 **9**	4 **2**	6 **4**
7 **5**	9 **7**	5 **3**
NE	N	NW

The Wood Snake Year

1
Monday

Animal: **Water Rooster**
Flying Star: **3**
Good Day: **Dragon**
Bad Day: **Rabbit**

2
Tuesday

Animal: **Wood Dog**
Flying Star: **2**
Good Day: **Rabbit**
Bad Day: **Dragon**

3
Wednesday

Animal: **Wood Pig**
Flying Star: **1**
Good Day: **Tiger**
Bad Day: **Snake**

4
Thursday

Animal: **Fire Rat**
Flying Star: **9**
Good Day: **Ox**
Bad Day: **Horse**

5
Friday

Animal: **Fire Ox**
Flying Star: **8**
Good Day: **Rat**
Bad Day: **Goat**

6
Saturday

Animal: **Earth Tiger**
Flying Star: **7**
Good Day: **Pig**
Bad Day: **Monkey**

7
Sunday

Animal: **Earth Rabbit**
Flying Star: **6**
Good Day: **Dog**
Bad Day: **Rooster**

SEPTEMBER MONTHLY CHINESE ZODIAC OVERVIEW

RAT

Energy stabilises this month, and projects will start to take shape. You'll gain clarity on your path to success, but financial stability remains uncertain. Stay vigilant with money matters, and strengthen your relationships with loved ones.

OX

September brings a mix of energies. Work will be demanding, but teamwork will lead to significant achievements. Spend quality time with loved ones, as relationships have the potential to improve. Prioritise self-care to avoid burnout.

TIGER

Although life may seem calm, underlying changes are forming. Be cautious with contracts and negotiations this month. Business owners should stick to traditional approaches. Protect your health by avoiding overexertion and staying grounded.

RABBIT

September's energy is better than last month's, though progress may be slow. Avoid rushing into deals and allow things to develop at their own pace. Stay optimistic and keep focused on long-term goals for the coming months.

DRAGON

September brings calm energy and emotional relief. Hard work will produce positive results, including improved income. To maintain well-being, focus on healthy eating to support your digestive system.

SNAKE

September brings optimistic energy, offering relief from recent stress. However, unexpected changes at work or in business could arise, so handle them with patience and focus. Stay firm in your decision-making process.

HORSE

Chaotic events may arise this month, so assess any problems carefully before taking action. Remain calm and avoid impulsive decisions, as they may worsen the situation. If travelling, take extra care of personal belongings to prevent losses.

The Wood Snake Year

8
Monday

Animal: **Metal Dragon**
Flying Star: **5**
Good Day: **Rooster**
Bad Day: **Dog**

9
Tuesday

Animal: **Metal Snake**
Flying Star: **4**
Good Day: **Monkey**
Bad Day: **Pig**

10
Wednesday

Animal: **Water Horse**
Flying Star: **3**
Good Day: **Goat**
Bad Day: **Rat**

11
Thursday

Animal: **Water Goat**
Flying Star: **2**
Good Day: **Horse**
Bad Day: **Ox**

12
Friday

Animal: **Wood Monkey**
Flying Star: **1**
Good Day: **Snake**
Bad Day: **Tiger**

13
Saturday

Animal: **Wood Rooster**
Flying Star: **9**
Good Day: **Dragon**
Bad Day: **Dog**

14
Sunday

Animal: **Fire Dog**
Flying Star: **8**
Good Day: **Rabbit**
Bad Day: **Dragon**

GOAT

September is a lucky and productive month. Creativity and fun will enhance your work. A new chapter in your personal life may begin, so be open to adjustments that lead to positive outcomes.

MONKEY

September's unstable energy requires careful management. Wealth energy will fluctuate, so avoid taking significant financial risks. Postpone major decisions until a more stable period.

ROOSTER

Positive energy continues, making this a busy month for business and social activities. Relationships will deepen and develop positively. Financial energy remains steady, supporting your endeavours.

DOG

Enter this month with a positive mindset to handle fluctuating energy. Give events time to unfold before making major plans. It's wise to delay significant decisions and focus on maintaining balance.

PIG

September's mixed energy requires flexibility. Financially, it is best to monitor your budget carefully and avoid big transactions. Focusing on home well-being will provide a strong foundation for future success.

15
Monday

Animal: **Fire Pig**
Flying Star: **7**
Good Day: **Tiger**
Bad Day: **Snake**

16
Tuesday

Animal: **Earth Rat**
Flying Star: **6**
Good Day: **Ox**
Bad Day: **Horse**

17
Wednesday

Animal: **Earth Ox**
Flying Star: **5**
Good Day: **Rat**
Bad Day: **Goat**

18
Thursday

Animal: **Metal Tiger**
Flying Star: **4**
Good Day: **Pig**
Bad Day: **Monkey**

19
Friday

Animal: **Metal Rabbit**
Flying Star: **3**
Good Day: **Dog**
Bad Day: **Rooster**

20
Saturday

Animal: **Water Dragon**
Flying Star: **2**
Good Day: **Rooster**
Bad Day: **Dog**

21
Sunday

Animal: **Water Snake**
Flying Star: **1**
Good Day: **Monkey**
Bad Day: **Pig**

ACTIVATING PEACH BLOSSOM LUCK FOR RELATIONSHIP & MARRIAGE LUCK

Individuals seeking to attract potential life partners for marriage can amplify their Peach Blossom Luck by incorporating their Peach Blossom Animal. This feng shui placement method is also an effective way to encourage your partner to step towards marriage!

Optimal Peach Blossom Enhancers are those embellished with symbols of love and marital joy. For instance, if you fall under the zodiac signs of Ox, Snake, or Rooster, consider placing a Peach Blossom Horse in the South. If your zodiac is Rat, Dragon, or Monkey, featuring a Peach Blossom Rooster in the West is advised.

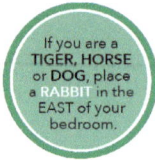

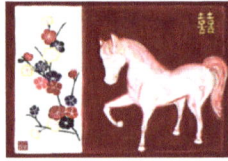

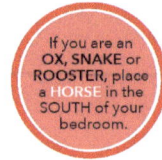

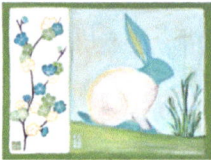

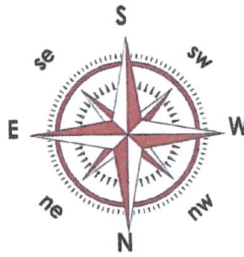

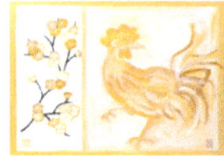

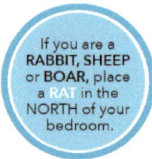

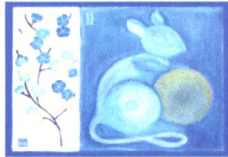

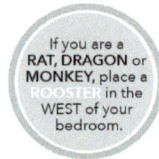

If you are a TIGER, HORSE or DOG, place a RABBIT in the EAST of your bedroom.

If you are an OX, SNAKE or ROOSTER, place a HORSE in the SOUTH of your bedroom.

If you are a RABBIT, SHEEP or BOAR, place a RAT in the NORTH of your bedroom.

If you are a RAT, DRAGON or MONKEY, place a ROOSTER in the WEST of your bedroom.

The Wood Snake Year

22
Monday

Animal: **Wood Horse**
Flying Star: **9**
Good Day: **Goat**
Bad Day: **Rat**
🔥 🪙

23
Tuesday

Animal: **Wood Goat**
Flying Star: **8**
Good Day: **Horse**
Bad Day: **Ox**

24
Wednesday

Animal: **Fire Monkey**
Flying Star: **7**
Good Day: **Snake**
Bad Day: **Tiger**
🪙

25
Thursday

Animal: **Fire Rooster**
Flying Star: **6**
Good Day: **Dragon**
Bad Day: **Dog**
✈️

26
Friday

Animal: **Earth Dog**
Flying Star: **5**
Good Day: **Rabbit**
Bad Day: **Dragon**
⚡✈️🪙🏎️🎬

27
Saturday

Animal: **Earth Pig**
Flying Star: **4**
Good Day: **Tiger**
Bad Day: **Snake**
🏠❤️🐷🥄✂️🎉

28
Sunday

Animal: **Metal Rat**
Flying Star: **3**
Good Day: **Ox**
Bad Day: **Horse**

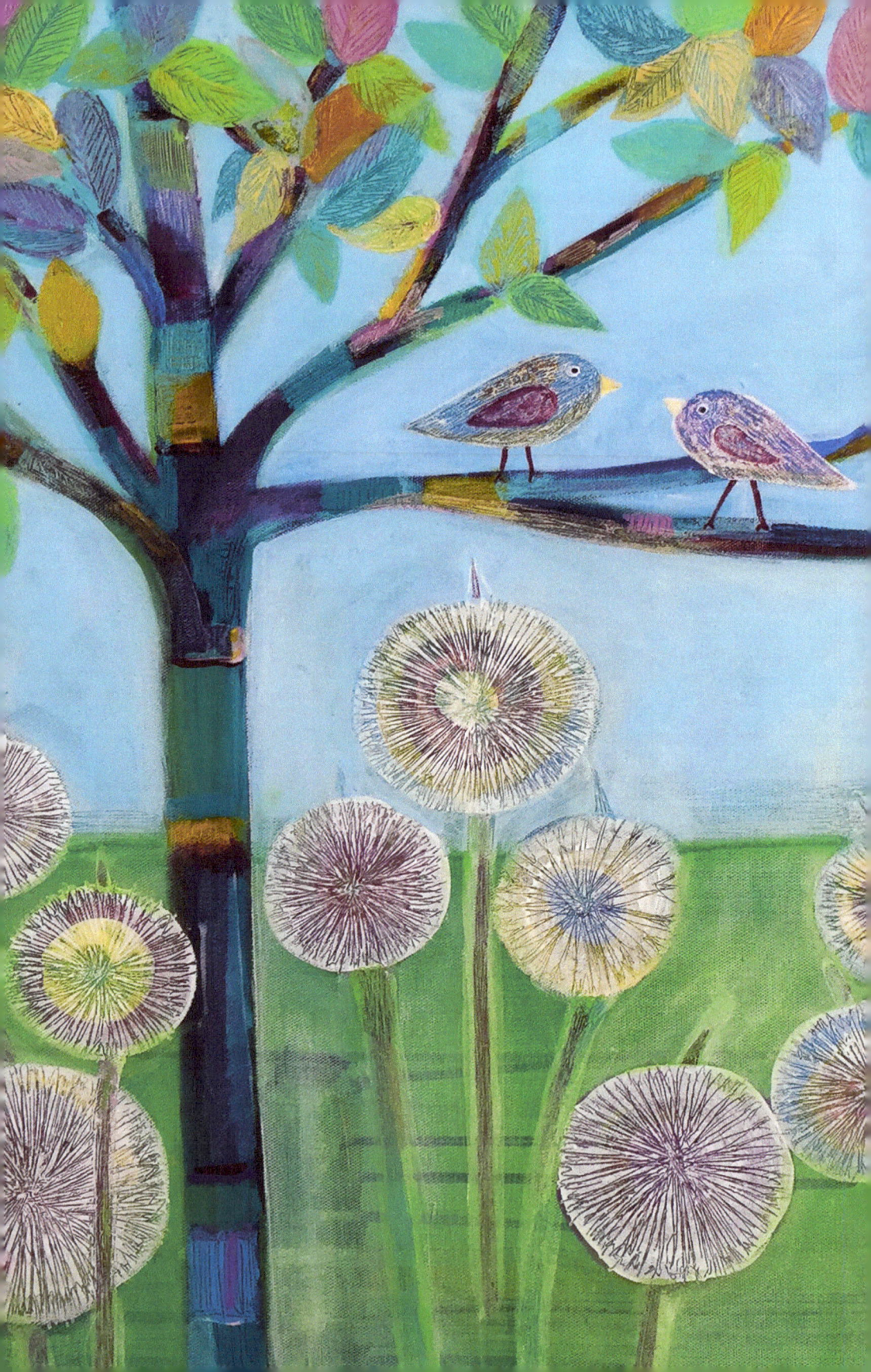

The Wood Snake Year

29 Monday	Animal: **Metal Ox** Flying Star: **2** Good Day: **Rat** Bad Day: **Goat**
30 Tuesday	Animal: **Water Tiger** Flying Star: **1** Good Day: **Pig** Bad Day: **Monkey**
1 Wednesday	Animal: **Water Rabbit** Flying Star: **9** Good Day: **Dog** Bad Day: **Dragon**
2 Thursday	Animal: **Wood Dragon** Flying Star: **8** Good Day: **Rooster** Bad Day: **Dog**
3 Friday	Animal: **Wood Snake** Flying Star: **7** Good Day: **Monkey** Bad Day: **Pig**
4 Saturday	Animal: **Fire Horse** Flying Star: **6** Good Day: **Goat** Bad Day: **Rat**
5 Sunday	Animal: **Fire Goat** Flying Star: **5** Good Day: **Horse** Bad Day: **Ox**

October 8 – November 6 is the Month of the Dog

Dog Chinese Horoscope 2025: Embracing Passion and Transformation

Dog Birth Years: 1922, 1934, 1946, 1958, 1970, 1982, 1994, 2006, 2018, 2030, 2042

In 2025, the Dog will experience the dynamic and transformative energy of the Yin Wood-Snake. This year brings a shift from the grounded and reliable Dragon of 2024 to a period marked by intensity and change, offering both challenges and opportunities.

Fire Snake Influence: Passion and Transformation

The Year of the Yin Wood Snake introduces intense energy and transformation for the Dog. This fiery and passionate influence encourages Dogs to embrace change, pursue new ventures, and channel their enthusiasm into personal and professional growth. The Fire Snake's energy will push Dogs to explore new opportunities and make bold decisions.

Career Focus: Bold Moves and Innovation

Professionally, the Fire Snake year presents opportunities for Dogs to make significant strides. This is a time for bold moves and innovative thinking. Embrace new projects and take calculated risks to advance your career. Networking and forming strategic partnerships will be crucial for success. Stay adaptable and open to new ideas to effectively navigate the changing professional landscape.

Love and Relationships: Intense and Transformative

In matters of the heart, the Fire Snake brings intensity and transformation. For single Dogs, this year offers exciting and potentially life-changing romantic prospects. Existing relationships may undergo profound changes, requiring open communication and a willingness to embrace new dynamics. Patience and understanding will maintain harmony in new and existing relationships.

Finance Strategies: Caution and Opportunity

Financially, the Year of the Fire Snake calls for cautious planning and strategic decision-making. While there are growth opportunities, avoid impulsive investments and focus on thorough research and long-term planning. Balancing enthusiasm with prudent financial management will help achieve stability and success.

Health and Well-being: Balancing Intensity

Maintaining health and well-being is essential with the Fire Snake's intense energy. Dogs should manage stress through relaxation techniques and ensure a balanced lifestyle with regular exercise and a nutritious diet. Engaging in mental and emotional respite activities will be necessary for overall health.

Symbolism of the Dog and Fire Snake: Passion and Transformation

The Dog's reliable and dedicated nature combines the Fire Snake's transformative and passionate influence in 2025. This year symbolises a period of significant change and growth. Dogs can achieve substantial personal and professional development by embracing the Fire Snake's dynamic energy.

2025: A Year of Dynamic Growth

The Year of the Yin Wood Snake offers Dogs a vibrant and transformative year. Embracing change, pursuing innovative opportunities, and maintaining a balanced approach to finances and health will help Dogs navigate the intense energy of 2025 successfully. With careful planning and adaptability, Dogs can turn challenges into opportunities for growth and success.

OCTOBER Flying Star 3, Discord, Conflict, and Caution

October begins the year under a cloud of discord as Flying Star 3 makes its ominous entrance into the celestial ballet. This star brings a surge of turbulent energies, vibrating with the unsettling resonance of conflict and strife. However, it's important to remember that there is potential for positive change even amid this turbulence. In its wake, seeds of gossip, disputes, and legal challenges find fertile ground, sprouting into full-blown turmoil. Far from benign, Flying Star 3 is a force of hostility, notorious for weaving a complex tapestry of violence, anger, and endless disagreements. It heralds a storm of misunderstandings, igniting fiery arguments and even litigation, casting a dark shadow over relationships between family members, friends, and colleagues.

The health ramifications that accompany this star are equally foreboding. It targets the liver, gallbladder, feet, and arms, manifesting in physical discomfort and malaise. As its influence spreads, productivity may falter, with the atmosphere thickening under the weight of conflict and friction.

Particularly vulnerable are those born in the Year of the Dog and Pig and the male head of the household. Marital bonds and familial harmony become entangled in the web of Flying Star 3's disruptive energies. The tension it fosters can cast a long shadow over relationships between spouses, eroding the foundations of stability within families and marriages. The looming threat of conflict with authorities and potential legal entanglements is a stark reminder of the need for heightened caution during this period. It's crucial to be alert and prepared, as this caution can help us navigate the challenges of Flying Star 3 with resilience and strength.

Under the influence of Flying Star 3, October demands a vigilant and defensive approach. However, it's important to remember that various remedies can counteract its negative energy. The traditional Chinese cure—a simple red piece of paper—can be a powerful tool to ward off its malign influence. Surroundings can be imbued with the protective energies of red and purple, introduced through decor, candles, and bright lights. The magic flaming wheel, a symbolic shield, can also be invoked to fend off negativity. Images of the fiery red phoenix or the watchful eagle can be guardians, defending against discord. For those seeking an extra layer of protection, the steadfast presence of temple lions and the vigilant gaze of the evil eye symbol can be enlisted, ensuring that the darkness remains at bay. These remedies offer a beacon of hope, empowering us to navigate the challenges of Flying Star 3 with resilience and strength.

In 2025, the Northwest sector will be particularly significant for feng shui enhancements. According to the Luo Shu or Bagua School of Feng Shui, this area is governed by the annual Flying Star 3, which symbolises critical figures such as the man of the house, influential benefactors, mentors, and supportive individuals. Focusing on this sector can strengthen personal and professional relationships, encouraging and motivating homeowners.

The Northwest is associated with the Metal element, which, in Chinese culture, signifies gold and family wealth. To harness and amplify this energy, incorporate metal décor items, objects in metallic colours, bells, or wind chimes. Additionally, placing a pair of noble elephants or the three Star Gods—representing health, wealth, and longevity—in the main living area can substantially benefit all household members, fostering a harmonious and prosperous environment.

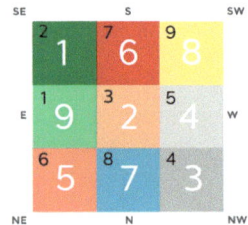

SE	S	SW
2 **1**	7 **6**	9 **8**
1 **9** E	3 **2**	5 **4** W
6 **5** NE	8 **7** N	4 **3** NW

The Wood Snake Year

6
Monday

Animal: **Earth Monkey**
Flying Star: **4**
Good Day: **Snake**
Bad Day: **Tiger**
✈ 🏠 ❤️ 🖤 🎬

7
Tuesday

Animal: **Earth Rooster**
Flying Star: **3**
Good Day: **Dragon**
Bad Day: **Rabbit**
✈

8
Wednesday

Animal: **Metal Dog**
Flying Star: **2**
Good Day: **Rabbit**
Bad Day: **Dragon**
✈ 🏠 💿

9
Thursday

Animal: **Metal Pig**
Flying Star: **1**
Good Day: **Tiger**
Bad Day: **Snake**
✈ 🏠

10
Friday

Animal: **Water Rat**
Flying Star: **9**
Good Day: **Ox**
Bad Day: **Horse**
🐾 💨 🎉

11
Saturday

Animal: **Water Ox**
Flying Star: **8**
Good Day: **Rat**
Bad Day: **Goat**

12
Sunday

Animal: **Wood Tiger**
Flying Star: **7**
Good Day: **Pig**
Bad Day: **Monkey**
🎬

OCTOBER MONTHLY CHINESE ZODIAC OVERVIEW

RAT

October's fluctuating energy may cause disruptions, so cautiously approach decisions, particularly financial ones. Some work projects may take longer to progress than expected. Make sure to take time for mental and emotional well-being, perhaps through relaxation or spending time with loved ones.

OX

October brings supportive energy. Maintaining a positive and happy outlook will boost your energy. Expect a busy month ahead with work keeping you occupied. Financially, avoid impulsive spending, as stability is critical to long-term success.

TIGER

After a few challenging months, the energy finally settles, giving you room to breathe and enjoy the flow. Work will go smoothly, and interpersonal issues will be resolved, making this an ideal time to socialise. New connections formed this month could benefit your professional life.

RABBIT

This is a busy month, but it may feel unproductive at work. Clear communication will be essential to navigate erratic energy. Rather than pushing for new achievements, review your progress and prepare for the upcoming year.

DRAGON

October's energy favours business networking and relationship building. Clear communication will be crucial for successful negotiations and presentations. While work is stable, avoid making significant changes or taking unnecessary risks this month.

SNAKE

Unstable energy this month means focusing on self-care is a priority. Therapeutic activities will help build confidence and restore balance. Travel and moving homes are indicated, but ensure that financial decisions are handled cautiously.

HORSE

October's unstable energy calls for careful management. Following established guidelines at work will benefit you. Make rest and a healthy lifestyle a priority to stay grounded and balanced amid the chaos.

The Wood Snake Year

13
Monday

Animal: **Wood Rabbit**
Flying Star: **6**
Good Day: **Dog**
Bad Day: **Dragon**

14
Tuesday

Animal: **Fire Dragon**
Flying Star: **5**
Good Day: **Rooster**
Bad Day: **Dog**

15
Wednesday

Animal: **Fire Snake**
Flying Star: **4**
Good Day: **Monkey**
Bad Day: **Pig**

16
Thursday

Animal: **Earth Horse**
Flying Star: **3**
Good Day: **Goat**
Bad Day: **Rat**

17
Friday

Animal: **Earth Goat**
Flying Star: **2**
Good Day: **Horse**
Bad Day: **Ox**

18
Saturday

Animal: **Metal Monkey**
Flying Star: **1**
Good Day: **Snake**
Bad Day: **Tiger**

19
Sunday

Animal: **Metal Rooster**
Flying Star: **9**
Good Day: **Dragon**
Bad Day: **Rabbit**

GOAT

This is a great time to start new projects, as positive energy will guide you. Maintain an open and flexible mindset to make the most of this month. Love relationships formed during this time are likely to be blissful and long-lasting.

MONKEY

October's energy is calmer, allowing you to refocus and maximise your potential. Work will proceed smoothly, and positive news is on the horizon. Make it a point to take a holiday and enjoy a vibrant social life.

ROOSTER

October may present challenges, especially at work. The energy is not supportive, which could impact your income. However, remain hopeful, as positive developments are on the horizon. Focus on handling current responsibilities efficiently.

DOG

Positive and harmonious energy is gaining momentum this month. Wealth energy is thriving, so financial gains are likely. New people entering your life will be supportive, and romance is in the air for singles. Some may even consider marriage.

PIG

October brings opportunities for personal development. Leverage your skills and take proactive steps toward achieving your goals. Financial energy is stable. Travel is indicated, but avoid risky activities such as mountain climbing or extreme sports to ensure safety.

The Wood Snake Year

20 Monday	Animal: **Water Dog** Flying Star: **8** Good Day: **Rabbit** Bad Day: **Dragon** ✈️🏠
21 Tuesday	Animal: **Water Pig** Flying Star: **7** Good Day: **Tiger** Bad Day: **Snake** ✈️🐒
22 Wednesday	Animal: **Wood Rat** Flying Star: **6** Good Day: **Ox** Bad Day: **Horse** 🐒
23 Thursday	Animal: **Wood Ox** Flying Star: **5** Good Day: **Rat** Bad Day: **Goat** ⚡
24 Friday	Animal: **Fire Tiger** Flying Star: **4** Good Day: **Pig** Bad Day: **Monkey** 🎬❤️🐖
25 Saturday	Animal: **Fire Rabbit** Flying Star: **3** Good Day: **Dog** Bad Day: **Dragon** ✈️🐚🎬
26 Sunday	Animal: **Earth Dragon** Flying Star: **2** Good Day: **Rooster** Bad Day: **Dog**

The Wood Snake Year

27
Monday

Animal: **Earth Snake**
Flying Star: **1**
Good Day: **Monkey**
Bad Day: **Pig**

28
Tuesday

Animal: **Metal Horse**
Flying Star: **9**
Good Day: **Goat**
Bad Day: **Rat**
✈️🏠🦽🔪💈🎞️

29
Wednesday

Animal: **Metal Goat**
Flying Star: **8**
Good Day: **Horse**
Bad Day: **Ox**
🐿️🏠

30
Thursday

Animal: **Water Monkey**
Flying Star: **7**
Good Day: **Snake**
Bad Day: **Tiger**
✈️🦽🎞️

31
Friday

Animal: **Water Rooster**
Flying Star: **6**
Good Day: **Dragon**
Bad Day: **Rabbit**
🏠🦽🎞️

1
Saturday

Animal: **Wood Dog**
Flying Star: **5**
Good Day: **Rabbit**
Bad Day: **Dragon**
⚡✈️

2
Sunday

Animal: **Wood Pig**
Flying Star: **4**
Good Day: **Tiger**
Bad Day: **Snake**
❤️👙✈️🏠

November 7 – December 6 is the Month of the Pig

Pig Chinese Horoscope 2025: Embracing Change and Transformation

Pig Birth Years: 1923, 1935, 1947, 1959, 1971, 1983, 1995, 2007, 2019, 2031, 2043

In 2025, the Pig will navigate the energetic and transformative influences of the Yin Wood-Snake. This year introduces a shift from the steady and reliable energies of the Dragon in 2024 to a period characterised by dynamic change and passion.

Fire Snake Influence: Transformation and Opportunity

The Year of the Yin Wood Snake brings an intense and transformative energy. For Pigs, this means a year of significant change, particularly in career and personal growth. The Fire Snake's influence encourages embracing new opportunities and taking bold steps towards transformation.

Career Focus: Embracing Innovation and Change

Professionally, the Fire Snake year presents a chance for Pigs to explore innovative ideas and adapt to changing circumstances. The dynamic energy of the Snake will push Pigs to step out of their comfort zones and pursue new career paths or projects. Focus on building new skills and forming strategic connections to advance your career. Be prepared for sudden changes and use them as opportunities for growth.

Love and Relationships: Intensity and Growth

The Fire Snake's energy brings passion and intensity to matters of the heart. Existing relationships may undergo profound changes, requiring open communication and a willingness to adapt. For single Pigs, exciting romantic possibilities are on the horizon. Approach new relationships with caution and mindfulness, ensuring you choose partners who align with your values and long-term goals.

Financial Strategies: Strategic Planning and Caution

Financially, the Year of the Fire Snake requires careful planning and strategic decision-making. While there are opportunities for financial growth, avoid impulsive investments and focus on thorough research. Embrace long-term financial strategies and seek expert advice to effectively navigate the changing economic landscape. Budgeting and prudent spending will be crucial for maintaining financial stability.

Health and Well-being: Balancing Intensity

The intense energy of the Fire Snake requires Pigs to maintain a balanced approach to health and well-being. Prioritise self-care by incorporating regular exercise, a nutritious diet, and effective stress management techniques into your routine. Engage in activities that promote mental and emotional well-being to balance the Fire Snake's dynamic influence.

Symbolism of the Pig and Fire Snake: Transformation and Passion

In 2025, the pig's nurturing and adaptable nature meets the Fire Snake's transformative and passionate energy. This combination symbolises a year of profound change and opportunity. By embracing the Fire Snake's vibrant energy, Pigs can achieve significant personal and professional development.

2025: A Year of Dynamic Change

The Year of the Yin Wood Snake offers Pigs a transformative and dynamic year. Embrace the opportunities for change and growth by adapting to new situations, pursuing innovative ideas, and maintaining a balanced approach to finances and health. With careful planning and an open mind, Pigs can turn challenges into opportunities for success and personal advancement.

NOVEMBER Flying Star 2: From Turmoil to Complex Energies

February ushers in the complex energies of Flying Star 2, a star that straddles both the remnants of its past and the promise of its future. As the cosmic dance continues, Star 2 takes place on the celestial stage, undergoing a profound metamorphosis that began in February 2024. While it now carries a glimmer of promising potential, the star's energy remains weak and still harbours the power of sickness and illness, a reminder of its turbulent legacy.

This transformation marks a significant shift in the cosmic landscape. Once a harbinger of affliction and negative energy during Period 8, Flying Star 2 is gradually shedding its inauspicious cloak as we progress into Period 9. Like a phoenix rising from the ashes, it embodies a new role as a force for positive change, although its influence remains cautious and tentative. Health and well-being, once threatened by this star, are now on the cusp of improvement, though the shadow of its past still lingers.

In Period 9, Flying Star 2 retains its Earth element, wielding energies that once wreaked havoc on health and peace. The early phases of this transition are marked by residual turbulence as the star's influence continues to present challenges, albeit less severe than in the past.

For 2025, Star 2's presence is felt in every home and building, casting a subtle but undeniable influence on the lives of those it touches. While there may be opportunities in property and real estate endeavours, these gains could come at the expense of health. The toll may be paid through illness or physical discomfort, underscoring the need to carefully manage this star's energy.

To harness Flying Star 2's transformative potential, a range of remedies is recommended. The Health Gourd, or Wu Lou, symbolises healing and well-being, best accompanied by Six Gold Coins on a vibrant red tassel. A Saltwater Cure can help neutralise lingering negative energies, while the presence of Quan Yin invites benevolent vibrations into space. Wearing a Wu Lou pendant or amulet is a protective talisman, particularly for those with low life force energy, shielding them from the star's lingering effects.

Metal elements play a crucial role in counteracting the challenges posed by Flying Star 2. Brass, copper, bronze, and pewter objects, artworks, and decor items introduce stability and balance into the environment. Incorporating white, silver, and gold shades further harmonises the space with the star's evolving energy in Period 9, aligning interiors with its subtle yet significant transformation.

In 2025, the annual Flying Star 2 will influence the Centre sector of the Luo Shu or Bagua School of Feng Shui. This sector is crucial for nurturing health and well-being, encompassing physical, emotional, and spiritual dimensions.

The centre of your home should remain open and unobstructed to ensure a healthy energy flow. Any blockages, such as those caused by staircases or bathrooms, can disrupt this flow. To counteract these issues, the area should be infused with the grounding energy of the Earth Element. Employ square shapes, earthy tones like yellow and tan, and materials such as ceramic tiles to restore balance and enhance vitality.

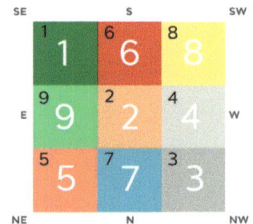

3
Monday

Animal: **Fire Rat**
Flying Star: **3**
Good Day: **Ox**
Bad Day: **Horse**
⌂☞✦🎉

4
Tuesday

Animal: **Fire Ox**
Flying Star: **2**
Good Day: **Rat**
Bad Day: **Goat**

5
Wednesday

Animal: **Earth Tiger**
Flying Star: **1**
Good Day: **Pig**
Bad Day: **Monkey**

6
Thursday

Animal: **Earth Rabbit**
Flying Star: **9**
Good Day: **Dog**
Bad Day: **Rooster**
✈⌂💰

7
Friday

Animal: **Metal Dragon**
Flying Star: **8**
Good Day: **Rooster**
Bad Day: **Dog**

8
Saturday

Animal: **Metal Snake**
Flying Star: **7**
Good Day: **Monkey**
Bad Day: **Pig**

9
Sunday

Animal: **Water Horse**
Flying Star: **6**
Good Day: **Goat**
Bad Day: **Rat**
✈⌂💰☞✦🎉🏛

NOVEMBER MONTHLY CHINESE ZODIAC OVERVIEW

RAT

You'll need extra effort to get things moving this month. Be wary of random money-making ideas, as they could lead to trouble. While business expansion is possible, achieving success may take more time and effort.

OX

November offers dynamic opportunities for growth. While challenges may arise, this is a chance to demonstrate resilience. Financially, the outlook is fair, so remain vigilant with spending and avoid unnecessary risks.

TIGER

Chaotic energy continues in November, so maintaining detachment and peace will benefit you. Surround yourself with supportive friends and take time to relax. Keep sports activities moderate to avoid injury or exhaustion.

RABBIT

This month's energy is slower than you might like, making it unsuitable for major changes. Practice patience and make the most of what you have. Financially, avoid excessive spending or impulsive investments.

DRAGON

November's calm and stable energy will bring emotional relief, but stress may still linger. If you're overwhelmed, consider taking a short holiday to regain balance and clarity.

SNAKE

Emotions may run high in November. Focus on staying optimistic and flexible. Walking, jogging, or drumming can help ground your energy and reduce stress. Don't let emotions cloud your decision-making.

HORSE

November may initially feel overwhelming, but you'll soon see progress in the right direction. Your joyful nature will help you make the most of the month. Manage finances carefully to ensure stability amidst the excitement.

The Wood Snake Year

10
Monday

Animal: **Water Goat**
Flying Star: **5**
Good Day: **Horse**
Bad Day: **Ox**
🐿️⚡

11
Tuesday

Animal: **Wood Monkey**
Flying Star: **4**
Good Day: **Snake**
Bad Day: **Tiger**
🧡🐍

12
Wednesday

Animal: **Wood Rooster**
Flying Star: **3**
Good Day: **Dragon**
Bad Day: **Rabbit**

13
Thursday

Animal: **Fire Dog**
Flying Star: **2**
Good Day: **Rabbit**
Bad Day: **Dragon**
🏰

14
Friday

Animal: **Fire Pig**
Flying Star: **1**
Good Day: **Tiger**
Bad Day: **Snake**

15
Saturday

Animal: **Earth Rat**
Flying Star: **9**
Good Day: **Ox**
Bad Day: **Horse**
✈️🏠💸🏰

16
Sunday

Animal: **Earth Ox**
Flying Star: **8**
Good Day: **Rat**
Bad Day: **Goat**
🐿️

GOAT

November's energy may cause dissatisfaction. Avoid making impulsive decisions that you might regret later. Focus on managing stress, staying grounded, and caring for your physical and mental health.

MONKEY

November is dominated by productive but unstable energy. Be prepared to act quickly when needed, but take time to assess situations carefully. People may be more sensitive, so ensure clear and compassionate communication to avoid misunderstandings.

ROOSTER

November's energy will accelerate rapidly, requiring efficiency and flexibility. Keep a close watch on self-care; managing stress will be crucial to maintaining well-being. Stay adaptable and patient through the month's fluctuations.

DOG

Positive, optimistic energy continues to build, boosting your finances. Investments are likely to yield gains, and business prospects are looking favourable. Use this momentum to move forward confidently.

PIG

November's energy is unstable, presenting both opportunities and challenges. Thorough planning will be needed for new projects or business ventures—Prioritise well-being and balance to navigate this unpredictable month successfully.

The Wood Snake Year

17
Monday

Animal: **Metal Tiger**
Flying Star: **7**
Good Day: **Pig**
Bad Day: **Monkey**
✈️🏠🍽️✂️💊🎉🎬

18
Tuesday

Animal: **Metal Rabbit**
Flying Star: **6**
Good Day: **Dog**
Bad Day: **Rooster**
✈️🏠🍽️✂️🎉

19
Wednesday

Animal: **Water Dragon**
Flying Star: **5**
Good Day: **Rooster**
Bad Day: **Dog**
🐀⚡

20
Thursday

Animal: **Water Snake**
Flying Star: **4**
Good Day: **Monkey**
Bad Day: **Pig**
❤️🖤

21
Friday

Animal: **Wood Horse**
Flying Star: **3**
Good Day: **Goat**
Bad Day: **Rat**
✈️🏠🍽️🎉🎬

22
Saturday

Animal: **Wood Goat**
Flying Star: **2**
Good Day: **Horse**
Bad Day: **Ox**

23
Sunday

Animal: **Fire Monkey**
Flying Star: **1**
Good Day: **Snake**
Bad Day: **Tiger**

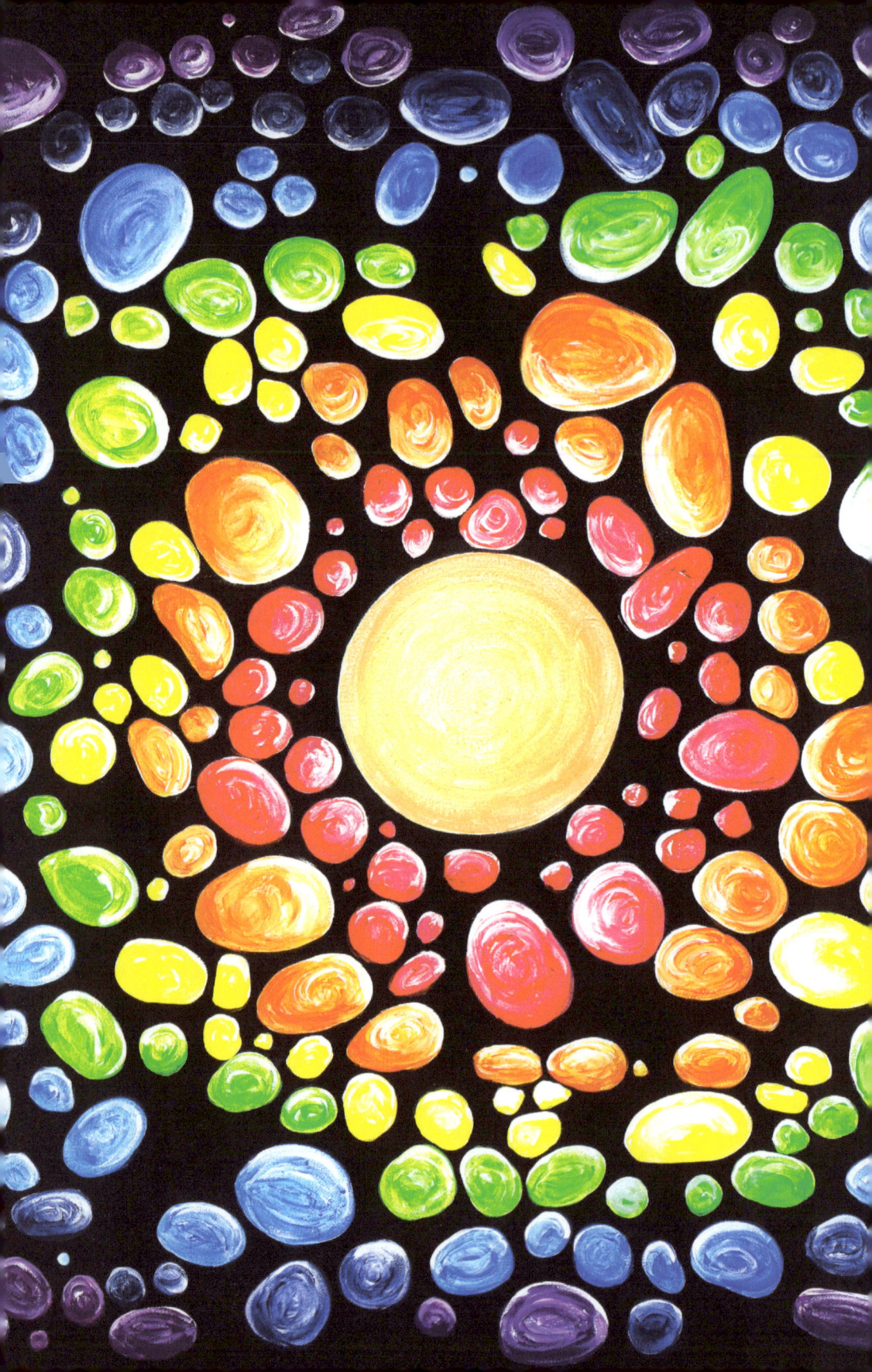

11 | NOVEMBER
2025

The Wood Snake Year

24
Monday

Animal: **Fire Rooster**
Flying Star: **9**
Good Day: **Dragon**
Bad Day: **Rabbit**
✈️🛞✏️🍴💥🎬

25
Tuesday

Animal: **Earth Dog**
Flying Star: **8**
Good Day: **Rabbit**
Bad Day: **Dragon**
🛞🎬

26
Wednesday

Animal: **Earth Pig**
Flying Star: **7**
Good Day: **Tiger**
Bad Day: **Snake**
✈️

27
Thursday

Animal: **Metal Rat**
Flying Star: **6**
Good Day: **Ox**
Bad Day: **Horse**
✈️🏠🛞✏️💥🎬

28
Friday

Animal: **Metal Ox**
Flying Star: **5**
Good Day: **Rat**
Bad Day: **Goat**
💃⚡🏠

29
Saturday

Animal: **Water Tiger**
Flying Star: **4**
Good Day: **Pig**
Bad Day: **Monkey**
✈️🏠❤️🥾🍴✏️💥🎬

30
Sunday

Animal: **Water Rabbit**
Flying Star: **3**
Good Day: **Dog**
Bad Day: **Rooster**
✈️🏠🛞🍴✏️🎬

December 7, 2024 - January 5, 2025: Month of the Rat

Rat Chinese Horoscope 2025: Embrace Change and Transformation

(1924, 1936, 1948, 1960, 1972, 1984, 1996, 2008, 2020)

The Year 2025 ushers in the dynamic and transformative energies of the Yin Wood-Snake. For Rats, this period brings both challenges and opportunities, marking a shift from the more stable influences of the previous year. Embrace the Fire Snake's vibrant energy to navigate significant changes and harness new potential.

Fire Snake Influence: Transformation and Passion

2025, the Rat will encounter the Yin Wood Snake's intense and transformative energy. The Fire Snake introduces a period of dynamic change, urging Rats to be adaptable and embrace innovation. This year is marked by a shift from stability to a time of passionate growth and transformation.

Career Outlook 2025: Innovation and Adaptation

The Fire Snake's influence will drive Rats to seek new career opportunities and adapt to evolving professional landscapes. This is a year to explore innovative ideas and take bold steps in your career. Competition may arise, but the Snake's energy will help Rats display their skills and reach their full potential. Focus on leveraging creativity and forming strategic connections to advance in your field.

Love and Relationships: Intensity and Growth

In the realm of love, 2025 brings both excitement and intensity. Existing relationships may undergo significant changes, requiring open communication and adaptability. For single Rats, the Fire Snake's influence offers new romantic possibilities with heightened passion. Approach new relationships with mindfulness, and ensure your connections align with your long-term goals. Married couples may experience a period of rekindled passion and deeper bonding.

Financial Outlook: Strategic Planning and Caution

Financially, the Year of the Fire Snake emphasises the need for careful planning and strategic decision-making. While there are opportunities for financial growth, avoid impulsive investments and focus on thorough research. Long-term financial strategies and prudent budgeting will be crucial for maintaining stability. Seek expert advice and be cautious with expenditures to ensure economic success.

Health and Wellness: Balancing Intensity

The dynamic energy of the Fire Snake calls for a balanced approach to health and well-being. Prioritise self-care by incorporating regular exercise, a nutritious diet, and effective stress management techniques into your routine. Engage in activities that promote mental and emotional well-being to counterbalance the Fire Snake's intense influence.

Symbolism of the Rat and Fire Snake: Transformation and Passion

In 2025, the rat's adaptable and resourceful nature meets the Fire Snake's transformative and passionate energy. This combination symbolises a year of significant change and opportunity. By embracing the Fire Snake's vibrant energy, Rats can achieve personal and professional growth.

2025: A Year of Dynamic Change

The Year of the Yin Wood Snake offers Rats a transformative and dynamic year. Embrace the opportunities for change and growth by adapting to new situations, pursuing innovative ideas, and maintaining a balanced approach to finances and health. With careful planning and an open mind, Rats can turn challenges into opportunities for success and advancement.

DECEMBER Flying Star 1: Triumph, Victory, and Brilliance

December brings forth the luminous energy of Flying Star 1, a beacon of positivity in the cosmic tapestry. Known as the Star of Triumph, this celestial force radiates its benevolent influence across fame, wealth, intelligence, and success. Its presence ushers in a season ripe for growth, achievement, and brilliance, casting a glow of opportunity over all who fall under its light.

With the guiding hand of Flying Star 1, individuals find themselves on pathways to triumph and victory. Its influence reaches far and wide, from elevating careers and reputations to enhancing status and recognition. This star particularly shines in career advancement and academic excellence, fuelling writing, research, and scholarly pursuits. In this celestial symphony, Flying Star 1 creates a harmonious environment where the seeds of success are sown and nurtured to fruition.

The optimism carried by this star is not fleeting; it lays the foundation for enduring triumphs. Whether overcoming competition, realising long-held dreams, or seizing wealth opportunities, the dynamic energy of Flying Star 1 fosters an atmosphere where influence and success flourish. Those aligned with this star, especially the eldest daughter and those born under the Dragon and Snake zodiacs, are encouraged to embrace challenges enthusiastically, knowing victory is within reach.

In addition to its career-enhancing qualities, Flying Star 1 offers a protective shield against health concerns, helping to bolster resilience and vitality. However, it also calls for mindfulness in navigating emotional turbulence. Maintaining emotional stability and guarding against depression is essential during this period, as the star's energy can amplify both positive and negative states.

Flying Star 1's elemental essence is Water, and it channels its triumph through this fluid and powerful conduit. Activating its potential involves introducing Yang energy, symbolised through metallic elements like wind chimes, collections of trophies, or medals that resonate with the star's victorious spirit. Flowing water features, such as fountains or a Victory Horse figurine accompanied by a Ruyi, further align the energies, paving the way for prosperity and success to flow effortlessly into your life.

In 2025, the annual Flying Star 1 will influence the Southeast sector of the Luo Shu or Bagua School of Feng Shui. Traditionally associated with wealth, prosperity, and financial growth, this sector offers fertile ground for enhancing income, cash flow, and overall economic success. It brings optimism and potential for monetary advancement, making it an area ripe for strategic Feng Shui adjustments.

The Southeast is governed by the Wood element, which thrives on the nurturing qualities of Water. To amplify the financial opportunities symbolised by Flying Star 1, enhance this sector with water-themed elements such as a water feature or a picturesque water image. Water strengthens the Wood energy and harmonises with green hues, plants, and floral decorations to further support financial luck. Ensure that the water flow is directed inward, enhancing the flow of prosperity into your home rather than allowing it to exit.

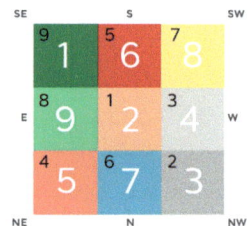

The Wood Snake Year

1
Monday

Animal: **Wood Dragon**
Flying Star: **2**
Good Day: **Rooster**
Bad Day: **Dog**
🪙 🏠 ✈

2
Tuesday

Animal: **Wood Snake**
Flying Star: **1**
Good Day: **Monkey**
Bad Day: **Pig**

3
Wednesday

Animal: **Fire Horse**
Flying Star: **9**
Good Day: **Goat**
Bad Day: **Rat**
🗳

4
Thursday

Animal: **Fire Goat**
Flying Star: **8**
Good Day: **Horse**
Bad Day: **Ox**
🗳

5
Friday

Animal: **Earth Monkey**
Flying Star: **7**
Good Day: **Snake**
Bad Day: **Tiger**

6
Saturday

Animal: **Earth Rooster**
Flying Star: **6**
Good Day: **Dragon**
Bad Day: **Rabbit**
🗳 🎉 ✈

7
Sunday

Animal: **Metal Dog**
Flying Star: **5**
Good Day: **Rabbit**
Bad Day: **Dragon**
🗳 ⚡

DECEMBER MONTHLY CHINESE ZODIAC OVERVIEW

RAT

Energy will accelerate in December, keeping you busy with work and activities. Amidst the hustle, make time for family and loved ones. Pay extra attention to the well-being of elderly family members, as they may need additional support during this busy season.

OX

December's vibrant and robust energy will bring a demanding pace. This is an excellent time for business networking and making new connections. However, prioritise self-care and nurture relationships with loved ones to maintain balance.

TIGER

December holds abundant and harmonious energy. You'll feel more positive and have new visions for the future. New job or business opportunities are likely to arise. Enjoy the festive season and not let work take over your personal life.

RABBIT

December will be busy and demanding. Focus is required to stay ahead of tasks and avoid conflicts at work. While business energy is optimistic, be extra careful with document errors and contracts.

DRAGON

December is filled with vibrant and optimistic energy. Work will remain busy, but take time to create new visions and goals for the year ahead. Financial aspects will improve, bringing a more prosperous outlook.

SNAKE

December's vibrant energy will boost your confidence and bring harmony to work and projects. It's important to be gentle with yourself and avoid negative influences. Surround yourself with supportive people to maintain your peace of mind.

HORSE

You're entering a more optimistic period, and most of your plans will proceed smoothly. Financial energy is vital, indicating extra income. Social energy is also high, allowing you to build and strengthen relationships quickly.

The Wood Snake Year

8
Monday

Animal: **Metal Pig**
Flying Star: **4**
Good Day: **Tiger**
Bad Day: **Snake**

9
Tuesday

Animal: **Water Rat**
Flying Star: **3**
Good Day: **Ox**
Bad Day: **Horse**

10
Wednesday

Animal: **Water Ox**
Flying Star: **2**
Good Day: **Rat**
Bad Day: **Goat**

11
Thursday

Animal: **Wood Tiger**
Flying Star: **1**
Good Day: **Pig**
Bad Day: **Monkey**

12
Friday

Animal: **Wood Rabbit**
Flying Star: **9**
Good Day: **Dog**
Bad Day: **Rooster**

13
Saturday

Animal: **Fire Dragon**
Flying Star: **8**
Good Day: **Rooster**
Bad Day: **Dog**

14
Sunday

Animal: **Fire Snake**
Flying Star: **7**
Good Day: **Monkey**
Bad Day: **Pig**

GOAT

December's energy is vibrant and optimistic, making it an excellent time to explore new ideas or projects. Creativity is high, leading to rewarding outcomes. There's also potential for financial gains if resources are managed wisely.

MONKEY

December is defined by fast-moving energy, so careful management is essential. Avoid making too many changes during this busy period. Business energy is strong, but remember to recharge with rest and relaxation to maintain well-being.

ROOSTER

December will be fulfilling and enriching. Expect new business opportunities early in the month, but stay grounded when finalising deals. Financial energy remains stable, setting the stage for a promising start to the new year.

DOG

Harmonious energy will bring a positive outlook in December. Wealth energy is rising, so watch your investments closely. Fun and adventure are on the horizon—embrace the festive spirit and enjoy yourself.

PIG

December's fast-paced energy will require you to go with the flow. Joyous celebrations will recharge your energy, so fully embrace the festive season. This month sets a positive tone for the upcoming Lunar New Year.

12 | DECEMBER
2025

The Wood Snake Year

15
Monday

Animal: **Earth Horse**
Flying Star: **6**
Good Day: **Goat**
Bad Day: **Rat**

16
Tuesday

Animal: **Earth Goat**
Flying Star: **5**
Good Day: **Horse**
Bad Day: **Ox**

🏭⚡

17
Wednesday

Animal: **Metal Monkey**
Flying Star: **4**
Good Day: **Snake**
Bad Day: **Tiger**

🥾❤️

18
Thursday

Animal: **Metal Rooster**
Flying Star: **3**
Good Day: **Dragon**
Bad Day: **Rabbit**

🐎

19
Friday

Animal: **Water Dog**
Flying Star: **2**
Good Day: **Rabbit**
Bad Day: **Dragon**

🏭

20
Saturday

Animal: **Water Pig**
Flying Star: **1**
Good Day: **Tiger**
Bad Day: **Snake**

21
Sunday

Animal: **Wood Rat**
Flying Star: **9/1**
Good Day: **Ox**
Bad Day: **Horse**

🚗

ACTIVATING FENG SHUI IN THE GARDEN

Each orientation possesses a distinct element. Employ the productive cycle to amplify the influence of each element. Utilise colours symbolically to manifest the essence of these elements.

SOUTH EAST	SOUTH	SOUTHWEST
The element of SMALL WOOD is associated with the colour light GREEN young growing plants, anything rectangular, the season of spring and expanding energy.	The element of FIRE is associated with the colour RED bright sunlight, the glow of lamps, anything sharp or pointed, the season of summer and upwards rising energy.	The element of BIG EARTH is associated with the colour OCHRE stones and pebbles, boulders and crystals, in between seasons and sideways moving energy.

EAST		WEST
The element of BIG WOOD is associated with the colour dark GREEN full grown plants, flowers and seeds, the season of spring and outwards flowing energy.	The CENTRE is of the EARTH ELEMENT	The element of SMALL METAL is associated with WHITE, GOLD & SILVER anything round and circular the season of autumn inward flowing energy.

NORTHEAST	NORTH	NORTHWEST
The element of SMALL EARTH is associated with the colour BEIGE the soil, the earth, anything square, in between seasons and horizontal moving energy.	The element of WATER is associated with the colours BLACK & BLUE anything wavy in shape, the season of winter and meandering energy.	The element of BIG METAL is associated with all METALLIC colours, GOLD & SILVER the season of autumn inward flowing energy.

The Wood Snake Year

22
Monday

Animal: **Wood Ox**
Flying Star: **2**
Good Day: **Rat**
Bad Day: **Goat**

23
Tuesday

Animal: **Fire Tiger**
Flying Star: **3**
Good Day: **Pig**
Bad Day: **Monkey**

24
Wednesday

Animal: **Fire Rabbit**
Flying Star: **4**
Good Day: **Dog**
Bad Day: **Rooster**

25
Thursday

Animal: **Earth Dragon**
Flying Star: **5**
Good Day: **Rooster**
Bad Day: **Dog**

26
Friday

Animal: **Earth Snake**
Flying Star: **6**
Good Day: **Monkey**
Bad Day: **Pig**

27
Saturday

Animal: **Metal Horse**
Flying Star: **7**
Good Day: **Goat**
Bad Day: **Rat**

28
Sunday

Animal: **Metal Goat**
Flying Star: **8**
Good Day: **Horse**
Bad Day: **Ox**

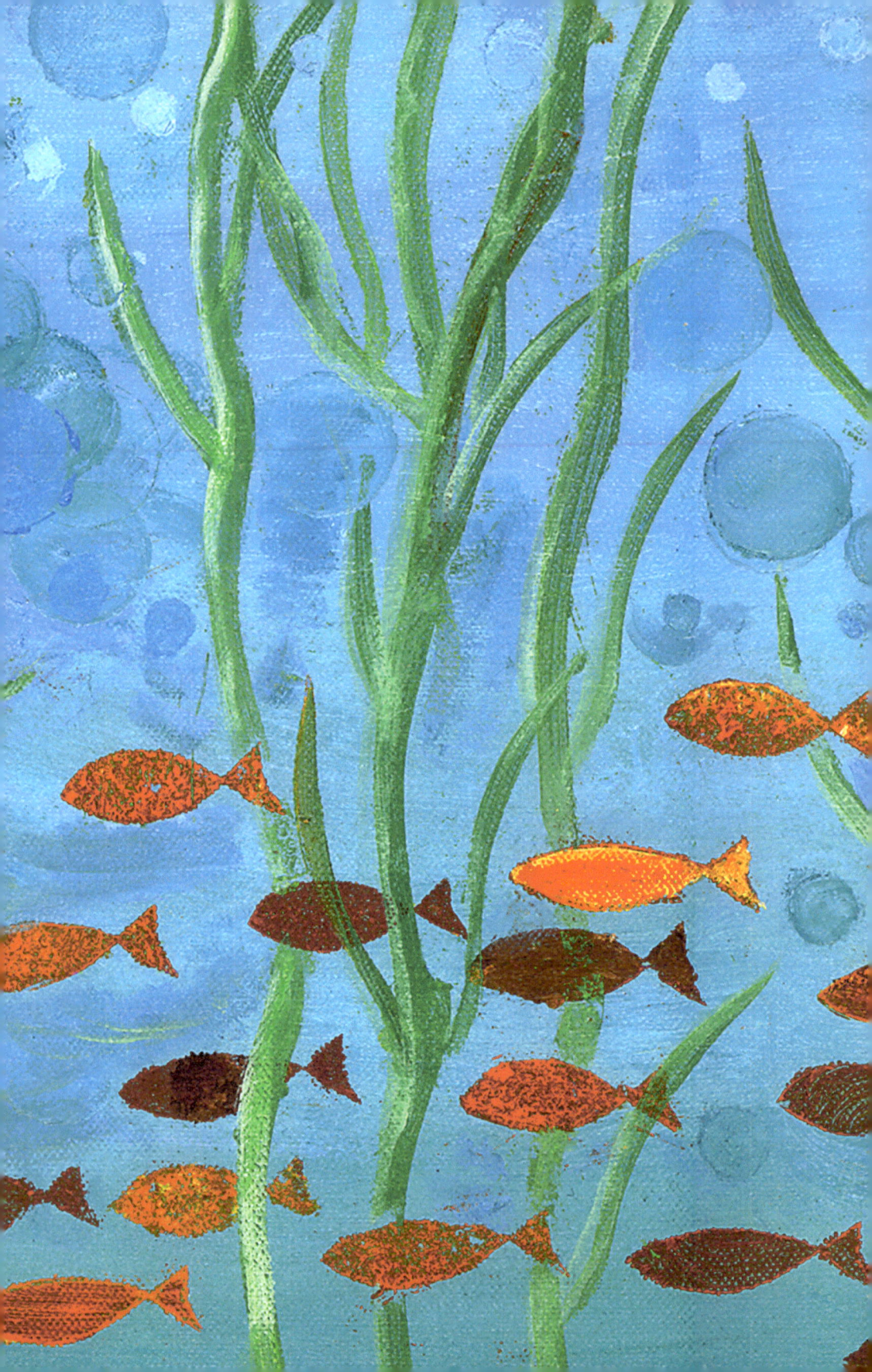

The Wood Snake Year

29
Monday

Animal: **Water Monkey**
Flying Star: **9**
Good Day: **Snake**
Bad Day: **Tiger**

💰🏠✈️

30
Tuesday

Animal: **Water Rooster**
Flying Star: **1**
Good Day: **Dragon**
Bad Day: **Rabbit**

🐿️

31
Wednesday (New Year Day)

Animal: **Wood Dog**
Flying Star: **2**
Good Day: **Rabbit**
Bad Day: **Dragon**

🎬

1
Thursday

Animal: **Wood Pig**
Flying Star: **3**
Good Day: **Tiger**
Bad Day: **Snake**

2
Friday

Animal: **Fire Rat**
Flying Star: **4**
Good Day: **Ox**
Bad Day: **Horse**

3
Saturday

Animal: **Fire Ox**
Flying Star: **5**
Good Day: **Rat**
Bad Day: **Goat**

⚡

4
Sunday

Animal: **Earth Tiger**
Flying Star: **6**
Good Day: **Pig**
Bad Day: **Monkey**

Your Kua Number

YEAR OF BIRTH	ANIMAL SIGN	HEAVENLY STEM	BORN BETWEEN...	MEN	WOMEN
1900	Rat	Metal	Jan 31, 1900-Feb 18, 1901	1	5
1901	Ox	Metal	Feb 19,1901 - Feb 7, 1902	9	6
1902	Tiger	Water	Feb 8, 1902-Jan 28, 1903	8	7
1903	Rabbit	Water	Jan 29,1903-Feb 28, 1904	7	8
1904	Dragon	Wood	Feb 16,1904- Feb 3,1905	6	9
1905	Snake	Wood	Feb 4, 1905-Jan 24, 1906	5	1
1906	Horse	Fire	Jan 25,1906-Feb 12,1907	4	2
1907	Goat	Fire	Feb 13, 1907- Feb 1, 1908	3	3
1908	Monkey	Earth	Feb 2,1908-Jan 21, 1909	2	4
1909	Rooster	Earth	Jan 22,1909- Feb 9,1910	1	5
1910	Dog	Metal	Feb 10, 1910-Jan 29,1911	9	6
1911	Pig	Metal	Jan 30,1911 - Feb 17,1912	8	7
1912	Rat	Water	Feb 18, 1912-Feb 5, 1913	7	8
1913	Ox	Water	Feb 6, 1913-Jan 25, 1914	6	9
1914	Tiger	Wood	Jan 26,1914- Feb 13, 1915	5	1
1915	Rabbit	Wood	Feb 14,1915-Feb 2,1916	4	2
1916	Dragon	Fire	Feb 3,1916-Jan 22,1917	3	3
1917	Snake	Fire	Jan 23, 1917- Feb 10, 1918	2	4
1918	Horse	Earth	Feb 11,1918-Jan 31, 1919	1	5
1919	Goat	Earth	Feb 1,1919-Feb 19, 1920	9	6
1920	Monkey	Metal	Feb 20, 1920-Feb 7, 1921	8	7
1921	Rooster	Metal	Feb 8,1921 - Jan 27, 1922	7	8
1922	Dog	Water	Jan 28, 1922-Feb 15, 1923	6	9
1923	Pig	Water	Feb 16,1923- Feb 4, 1924	5	1
1924	Rat	Wood	Feb 5, 1924-Jan 23, 1925	4	2
1925	Ox	Wood	Jan 24, 1925- Feb 12, 1926	3	3
1926	Tiger	Fire	Feb 13,1926- Feb 1,1927	2	4
1927	Rabbit	Fire	Feb 2, 1927-Jan 22, 1928	1	5

YEAR OF BIRTH	ANIMAL SIGN	HEAVENLY STEM	BORN BETWEEN...	MEN	WOMEN
1928	Dragon	Earth	Jan 23,1928- Feb 9, 1929	9	6
1929	Snake	Earth	Feb 10,1929 - Jan 29,1930	8	7
1930	Horse	Metal	Jan 30,1930- Feb 16 1931	7	8
1931	Goat	Metal	Feb 17,1931 - Feb 5, 1932	6	9
1932	Monkey	Water	Feb 6, 1932-Jan 25,1933	5	1
1933	Rooster	Water	Jan 26, 1933-Feb 13, 1934	4	2
1934	Dog	Wood	Feb 14,1934- Feb 3,1935	3	3
1935	Pig	Wood	Feb 4, 1935-Jan 23, 1936	2	4
1936	Rat	Fire	Jan 24, 1936- Feb 10,1937	1	5
1937	Ox	Fire	Feb 11,1937-Jan 30,1938	9	6
1938	Tiger	Earth	Jan 31,1938-Feb 18, 1939	8	7
1939	Rabbit	Earth	Feb 19, 1939- Feb 7, 1940	7	8
1940	Dragon	Metal	Feb 8, 1940-Jan 26, 1941	6	9
1941	Snake	Metal	Jan 27, 1941 - Feb 14, 1942	5	1
1942	Horse	Water	Feb 15, 1942 - Feb 4,1943	4	2
1943	Goat	Water	Feb 5, 1943-Jan 24, 1944	3	3
1944	Monkey	Wood	Jan 25,1944-Feb 12,1945	2	4
1945	Rooster	Wood	Feb 13, 1945 - Feb 1, 1946	1	5
1946	Dog	Fire	Feb 2, 1946-Jan 21, 1947	9	6
1947	Pig	Fire	Jan 22, 1947-Feb 9, 1948	8	7
1948	Rat	Earth	Feb 10, 1948-Jan 28, 1949	7	8
1949	Ox	Earth	Jan 29, 1949-Feb 16, 1950	6	9
1950	Tiger	Metal	Feb 17 1950- Feb 5,1951	5	1
1951	Rabbit	Metal	Feb 6, 1951 - Jan 26 1952	4	2
1952	Dragon	Water	Jan 27,1952 - Feb 13,1953	3	3
1953	Snake	Water	Feb 14, 1953- Feb 2, 1954	2	4
1954	Horse	Wood	Feb 3, 1954-Jan 23, 1955	1	5
1955	Goat	Wood	Jan 24, 1955-Feb 11, 1956	9	6
1956	Monkey	Fire	Feb 12,1956-Jan 30, 1957	8	7
1957	Rooster	Fire	Jan 31, 1957-Feb 17, 1958	7	8
1958	Dog	Earth	Feb 18, 1958-Feb 7 1959	6	9
1959	Pig	Earth	Feb 8, 1959-Jan 27, 1960	5	1

YEAR OF BIRTH	ANIMAL SIGN	HEAVENLY STEM	BORN BETWEEN...	MEN	WOMEN
1960	Rat	Metal	Jan 28, 1960 - Feb 14, 1961	4	2
1961	Ox	Metal	Feb 15, 1961 - Feb 4, 1962	3	3
1962	Tiger	Water	Feb 5, 1962 - Jan 24, 1963	2	4
1963	Rabbit	Water	Jan 25, 1963- Feb 12 1964	1	5
1964	Dragon	Wood	Feb 13, 1964-Feb 1,1965	9	6
1965	Snake	Wood	Feb 2, 1965-Jan 20, 1966	8	7
1966	Horse	Fire	Jan 21,1966-Feb 8,1967	7	8
1967	Goat	Fire	Feb 9,1967-Jan 29,1968	6	9
1968	Monkey	Earth	Jan 30, 1968-Feb 16, 1969	5	1
1969	Rooster	Earth	Feb 17, 1969-Feb 5, 1970	4	2
1970	Dog	Metal	Feb 6, 1970-Jan 26,1971	3	3
1971	Pig	Metal	Jan 27, 1971 - Feb 14, 1972	2	4
1972	Rat	Water	Feb 15, 1972-Feb 2, 1973	1	5
1973	Ox	Water	Feb 3, 1973-Jan 22, 1974	9	6
1974	Tiger	Wood	Jan 23, 1974-Feb 10, 1975	8	7
1975	Rabbit	Wood	Feb 11, 1975 - Jan 30, 1976	7	8
1976	Dragon	Fire	Jan 31, 1976-Feb 17 1977	6	9
1977	Snake	Fire	Feb 18,1977- Feb 6, 1978	5	1
1978	Horse	Earth	Feb 7, 1978 - Jan 27, 1979	4	2
1979	Goat	Earth	Jan 28, 1979 - Feb 15, 1980	3	3
1980	Monkey	Metal	Feb 16, 1980- Feb 4, 1981	2	4
1981	Rooster	Metal	Feb 5, 1981 - Jan 24, 1982	1	5
1982	Dog	Water	Jan 25, 1982-Feb12, 1983	9	6
1983	Pig	Water	Feb 13,1983- Feb 1,1984	8	7
1984	Rat	Wood	Feb 2,1984- Feb 19, 1985	7	8
1985	Ox	Wood	Feb 20, 1985-Feb 8, 1986	6	9
1986	Tiger	Fire	Feb 9, 1986-Jan 28, 1987	5	1
1987	Rabbit	Fire	Jan 29, 1987- Feb 16, 1988	4	2
1988	Dragon	Earth	Feb 17, 1988- Feb 5, 1989	3	3
1989	Snake	Earth	Feb 6, 1989-Jan 26, 1990	2	4
1990	Horse	Metal	Jan 27,1990 - Feb 14,1991	1	5
1991	Goat	Metal	Feb 15, 1991 - Feb 3, 1992	9	6

YEAR OF BIRTH	ANIMAL SIGN	HEAVENLY STEM	BORN BETWEEN...	MEN	WOMEN
1992	Monkey	Water	Feb 4, 1992-Jan 22, 1993	8	7
1993	Rooster	Water	Jan 23,1993 - Feb 9, 1994	7	8
1994	Dog	Wood	Feb 10, 1994-Jan 30, 1995	6	9
1995	Pig	Wood	Jan 31, 1995-Feb 18, 1996	5	1
1996	Rat	Fire	Feb 19, 1996 - Feb 6, 1997	4	2
1997	Ox	Fire	Feb 7, 1997 - Jan 27, 1998	3	3
1998	Tiger	Earth	Jan 28, 1998 - Feb 15,1999	2	4
1999	Rabbit	Earth	Feb 16, 1999-Feb 4, 2000	1	5
2000	Dragon	Metal	Feb 5, 2000 - Jan 23, 2001	9	6
2001	Snake	Metal	Jan 24, 2001 - Feb 11,2002	8	7
2002	Horse	Water	Feb 12, 2002-Jan 31,2003	7	8
2003	Goat	Water	Feb 1,2003 - Jan 21,2004	6	9
2004	Monkey	Wood	Jan 22, 2004 - Feb 8, 2005	5	1
2005	Rooster	Wood	Feb 9, 2005 - Jan 28, 2006	4	2
2006	Dog	Fire	Jan 29, 2006-Feb 17 2007	3	3
2007	Pig	Fire	Feb 18, 2007 - Feb 6, 2008	2	4
2008	Rat	Earth	Feb 7 2008 - Jan 25, 2009	1	5
2009	Ox	Earth	Jan 26, 2009 - Feb 13, 2010	9	6
2010	Tiger	Metal	Feb 14, 2010-Feb 2, 2011	8	7
2011	Rabbit	Metal	Feb 3, 2011 - Jan 22, 2012	7	8
2012	Dragon	Water	Jan 23, 2012-Feb 9, 2013	6	9
2013	Snake	Water	Feb 10, 2013-Jan 30, 2014	5	1
2014	Horse	Wood	Jan 31,2014-Feb 18, 2015	4	2
2015	Goat	Wood	Feb 19, 2015-Feb 7, 2016	3	3
2016	Monkey	Fire	Feb 8, 2016-Jan 27,2017	2	4
2017	Rooster	Fire	Jan 28, 2017-Feb 15, 2018	1	5
2018	Dog	Earth	Feb 16, 2018-Feb 4, 2019	9	6
2019	Pig	Earth	Feb 5, 2019 - Jan 24, 2020	8	7
2020	Rat	Metal	Jan 25, 2020 - Feb 11,2021	7	8
2021	Ox	Metal	Feb 12, 2021 - Jan 31,2022	6	9
2022	Tiger	Water	Feb 1,2022-Jan 21,2023	5	1
2023	Rabbit	Water	Jan 22, 2023 - Feb 9, 2024	4	2

YEAR OF BIRTH	ANIMAL SIGN	HEAVENLY STEM	BORN BETWEEN...	MEN	WOMEN
2024	Dragon	Wood	Feb 10, 2024-Jan 28, 2025	3	3
2025	Snake	Wood	Jan 29, 2025-Feb 16, 2026	2	4
2026	Horse	Fire	Feb 17, 2026 - Feb 5, 2027	1	5
2027	Goat	Fire	Feb 6, 2027 - Jan 25, 2028	9	6
2028	Monkey	Earth	Jan 26, 2028 - Feb 12, 2029	8	7
2029	Rooster	Earth	Feb 13, 2029-Feb 2, 2030	7	8
2030	Dog	Metal	Feb 3, 2030 - Jan 22, 2031	6	9
2031	Pig	Metal	Jan 23, 2031 - Feb 10, 2032	5	1
2032	Rat	Water	Feb 11,2032-Jan 30, 2033	4	2
2033	Ox	Water	Jan 31,2033- Feb 18, 2034	3	3
2034	Tiger	Wood	Feb 19, 2034 - Feb 7 2035	2	4
2035	Rabbit	Wood	Feb 8, 2035 - Jan 27, 2036	1	5
2036	Dragon	Fire	Jan 28, 2036 - Feb 14, 2037	9	6
2037	Snake	Fire	Feb 15, 2037- Feb 3, 2038	8	7
2038	Horse	Earth	Feb 4, 2038 - Jan 23, 2039	7	8
2039	Goat	Earth	Jan 24, 2039 - Feb 11,2040	6	9
2040	Monkey	Metal	Feb 12, 2040-Jan 31,2041	5	1
2041	Rooster	Metal	Feb 1,2041 - Jan 21,2042	4	2
2042	Dog	Water	Jan 22, 2042 - Feb 9, 2043	3	3
2043	Pig	Water	Feb 10, 2043-Jan 29,2044	2	4
2044	Rat	Wood	Jan 30, 2044-Feb 16, 2045	1	5
2045	Ox	Wood	Feb 17 2045 - Feb 5, 2046	9	6
2046	Tiger	Fire	Feb 6, 2046 - Jan 25, 2047	8	7
2047	Rabbit	Fire	Jan 26, 2047 - Feb 13, 2048	7	8
2048	Dragon	Earth	Feb 14, 2048 - Feb 1,2049	6	9
2049	Snake	Earth	Feb 2, 2049 - Jan 22, 2050	5	1
2050	Horse	Metal	Jan 23, 2050 - Feb 11,2051	4	2
2051	Goat	Metal	Feb 12, 2051 - Jan 31,2052	3	3
2052	Monkey	Water	Feb 1,2052-Feb 18, 2053	2	4
2053	Rooster	Water	Feb 19, 2053 - Feb 7, 2054	1	5
2054	Dog	Wood	Feb 8, 2054 - Jan 27, 2055	9	6

Auspicious and Inauspicious Directions
Based on your Kua Number

Position yourself in a favourble orientation for significant activities. Whether seating a deal, engaging in work or meals, delivering a presentation, attending a learning session, or even during sleep, ensure your head is directed towards a positive angle. Steer clear of unfavourable orientations whenever possible.

Auspicious Directions:

Kua Number	Sheng Chi (Best Direction)	Tien Yi (Health Direction)	Nien Yen (Romance Direction)	Fu Wei (Personal Growth Direction)
1	Southeast	East	South	North
2	Northeast	West	Northwest	Southwest
3	South	North	Southeast	East
4	North	South	East	Southeast
6	West	Northeast	Southwest	Northwest
7	Northwest	Southwest	Northeast	West
8	Southwest	Northwest	West	Northeast
9	East	Southeast	North	South

Inauspicious Directions:

Kua Number	Ho Hai (Unlucky)	Wu Kwei (Five Ghosts)	Lui Sha (Six Killings)	Chueh Ming (Total Loss)
1	West	Northeast	Northwest	Southwest
2	East	Southeast	South	North
3	Southwest	Northwest	Northeast	West
4	Northwest	Southwest	West	Northeast
6	Southeast	East	North	South
7	North	South	Southeast	East
8	South	North	East	Southeast
9	Northeast	West	Southwest	Northwest

2025

JANUARY

MO		6	13	20	27
TU		7	14	21	28
WE	1	8	15	22	29
TH	2	9	16	23	30
FR	3	10	17	24	31
SA	4	11	18	25	
SU	5	12	19	26	

FEBRUARY

MO		3	10	17	24
TU		4	11	18	25
WE		5	12	19	26
TH		6	13	20	27
FR		7	14	21	28
SA	1	8	15	22	
SU	2	9	16	23	

MARCH

MO	31	3	10	17	24
TU		4	11	18	25
WE		5	12	19	26
TH		6	13	20	27
FR		7	14	21	28
SA	1	8	15	22	29
SU	2	9	16	23	30

APRIL

MO		7	14	21	28
TU	1	8	15	22	29
WE	2	9	16	23	30
TH	3	10	17	24	
FR	4	11	18	25	
SA	5	12	19	26	
SU	6	13	20	27	

MAY

MO		5	12	19	26
TU		6	13	20	27
WE		7	14	21	28
TH	1	8	15	22	29
FR	2	9	16	23	30
SA	3	10	17	24	31
SU	4	11	18	25	

JUNE

MO	30	2	9	16	23
TU		3	10	17	24
WE		4	11	18	25
TH		5	12	19	26
FR		6	13	20	27
SA		7	14	21	28
SU	1	8	15	22	29

JULY

MO		7	14	21	28
TU	1	8	15	22	29
WE	2	9	16	23	30
TH	3	10	17	24	31
FR	4	11	18	25	
SA	5	12	19	26	
SU	6	13	20	27	

AUGUST

MO		4	11	18	25
TU		5	12	19	26
WE		6	13	20	27
TH		7	14	21	28
FR	1	8	15	22	29
SA	2	9	16	23	30
SU	3	10	17	24	31

SEPTEMBER

MO	1	8	15	22	29
TU	2	9	16	23	30
WE	3	10	17	24	
TH	4	11	18	25	
FR	5	12	19	26	
SA	6	13	20	27	
SU	7	14	21	28	

OCTOBER

MO		6	13	20	27
TU		7	14	21	28
WE	1	8	15	22	29
TH	2	9	16	23	30
FR	3	10	17	24	31
SA	4	11	18	25	
SU	5	12	19	26	

NOVEMBER

MO		3	10	17	24
TU		4	11	18	25
WE		5	12	19	26
TH		6	13	20	27
FR		7	14	21	28
SA	1	8	15	22	29
SU	2	9	16	23	30

DECEMBER

MO	1	8	15	22	29
TU	2	9	16	23	30
WE	3	10	17	24	31
TH	4	11	18	25	
FR	5	12	19	26	
SA	6	13	20	27	
SU	7	14	21	28	

2026

JANUARY
MO		5	12	19	26
TU		6	13	20	27
WE		7	14	21	28
TH	1	8	15	22	29
FR	2	9	16	23	30
SA	3	10	17	24	31
SU	4	11	18	25	

FEBRUARY
MO		2	9	16	23
TU		3	10	17	24
WE		4	11	18	25
TH		5	12	19	26
FR		6	13	20	27
SA		7	14	21	28
SU	1	8	15	22	

MARCH
MO	30	2	9	16	23
TU	31	3	10	17	24
WE		4	11	18	25
TH		5	12	19	26
FR		6	13	20	27
SA		7	14	21	28
SU	1	8	15	22	29

APRIL
MO		6	13	20	27
TU		7	14	21	28
WE	1	8	15	22	29
TH	2	9	16	23	30
FR	3	10	17	24	
SA	4	11	18	25	
SU	5	12	19	26	

MAY
MO		4	11	18	25
TU		5	12	19	26
WE		6	13	20	27
TH		7	14	21	28
FR	1	8	15	22	29
SA	2	9	16	23	30
SU	3	10	17	24	31

JUNE
MO	1	8	15	22	29
TU	2	9	16	23	30
WE	3	10	17	24	
TH	4	11	18	25	
FR	5	12	19	26	
SA	6	13	20	27	
SU	7	14	21	28	

JULY
MO		6	13	20	27
TU		7	14	21	28
WE	1	8	15	22	29
TH	2	9	16	23	30
FR	3	10	17	24	31
SA	4	11	18	25	
SU	5	12	19	26	

AUGUST
MO	31	3	10	17	24
TU		4	11	18	25
WE		5	12	19	26
TH		6	13	20	27
FR		7	14	21	28
SA	1	8	15	22	29
SU	2	9	16	23	30

SEPTEMBER
MO		7	14	21	28
TU	1	8	15	22	29
WE	2	9	16	23	30
TH	3	10	17	24	
FR	4	11	18	25	
SA	5	12	19	26	
SU	6	13	20	27	

OCTOBER
MO		5	12	19	26
TU		6	13	20	27
WE		7	14	21	28
TH	1	8	15	22	29
FR	2	9	16	23	30
SA	3	10	17	24	31
SU	4	11	18	25	

NOVEMBER
MO	30	2	9	16	23
TU		3	10	17	24
WE		4	11	18	25
TH		5	12	19	26
FR		6	13	20	27
SA		7	14	21	28
SU	1	8	15	22	29

DECEMBER
MO		7	14	21	28
TU	1	8	15	22	29
WE	2	9	16	23	30
TH	3	10	17	24	31
FR	4	11	18	25	
SA	5	12	19	26	
SU	6	13	20	27	

2025 Year Planner

DAY	JANUARY	FEBRUARY	MARCH
MONDAY	1		
TUESDAY	2		
WEDNESDAY	3		
THURSDAY	4	1	
FRIDAY	5	2	1
SATURDAY	6	3	2
SUNDAY	7	4	3
MONDAY	8	5	4
TUESDAY	9	6	5
WEDNESDAY	10	7	6
THURSDAY	11	8	7
FRIDAY	12	9	8
SATURDAY	13	10	9
SUNDAY	14	11	10
MONDAY	15	12	11
TUESDAY	16	13	12
WEDNESDAY	17	14	13
THURSDAY	18	15	14
FRIDAY	19	16	15
SATURDAY	20	17	16
SUNDAY	21	18	17
MONDAY	22	19	18
TUESDAY	23	20	19
WEDNESDAY	24	21	20
THURSDAY	25	22	21
FRIDAY	26	23	22
SATURDAY	27	24	23
SUNDAY	28	25	24
MONDAY	29	26	25
TUESDAY	30	27	26
WEDNESDAY	31	28	27
THURSDAY		29	28
FRIDAY			29
SATURDAY			30
SUNDAY			31
MONDAY			
TUESDAY			

2025 Year Planner

APRIL	MAY	JUNE	DAY
1			MONDAY
2			TUESDAY
3	1		WEDNESDAY
4	2		THURSDAY
5	3		FRIDAY
6	4	1	SATURDAY
7	5	2	SUNDAY
8	6	3	MONDAY
9	7	4	TUESDAY
10	8	5	WEDNESDAY
11	9	6	THURSDAY
12	10	7	FRIDAY
13	11	8	SATURDAY
14	12	9	SUNDAY
15	13	10	MONDAY
16	14	11	TUESDAY
17	15	12	WEDNESDAY
18	16	13	THURSDAY
19	17	14	FRIDAY
20	18	15	SATURDAY
21	19	16	SUNDAY
22	20	17	MONDAY
23	21	18	TUESDAY
24	22	19	WEDNESDAY
25	23	20	THURSDAY
26	24	21	FRIDAY
27	25	22	SATURDAY
28	26	23	SUNDAY
29	27	24	MONDAY
30	28	25	TUESDAY
	29	26	WEDNESDAY
	30	27	THURSDAY
	31	28	FRIDAY
		29	SATURDAY
		30	SUNDAY
			MONDAY
			TUESDAY

2025 Year Planner

DAY	JULY	AUGUST	SEPTEMBER
MONDAY	1		
TUESDAY	2		
WEDNESDAY	3		
THURSDAY	4	1	
FRIDAY	5	2	
SATURDAY	6	3	
SUNDAY	7	4	1
MONDAY	8	5	2
TUESDAY	9	6	3
WEDNESDAY	10	7	4
THURSDAY	11	8	5
FRIDAY	12	9	6
SATURDAY	13	10	7
SUNDAY	14	11	8
MONDAY	15	12	9
TUESDAY	16	13	10
WEDNESDAY	17	14	11
THURSDAY	18	15	12
FRIDAY	19	16	13
SATURDAY	20	17	14
SUNDAY	21	18	15
MONDAY	22	19	16
TUESDAY	23	20	17
WEDNESDAY	24	21	18
THURSDAY	25	22	19
FRIDAY	26	23	20
SATURDAY	27	24	21
SUNDAY	28	25	22
MONDAY	29	26	23
TUESDAY	30	27	24
WEDNESDAY	31	28	25
THURSDAY		29	26
FRIDAY		30	27
SATURDAY		31	28
SUNDAY			29
MONDAY			30
TUESDAY			

2025 Year Planner

OCTOBER	NOVEMBER	DECEMBER	DAY
			MONDAY
1			TUESDAY
2			WEDNESDAY
3			THURSDAY
4	1		FRIDAY
5	2		SATURDAY
6	3	1	SUNDAY
7	4	2	MONDAY
8	5	3	TUESDAY
9	6	4	WEDNESDAY
10	7	5	THURSDAY
11	8	6	FRIDAY
12	9	7	SATURDAY
13	10	8	SUNDAY
14	11	9	MONDAY
15	12	10	TUESDAY
16	13	11	WEDNESDAY
17	14	12	THURSDAY
18	15	13	FRIDAY
19	16	14	SATURDAY
20	17	15	SUNDAY
21	18	16	MONDAY
22	19	17	TUESDAY
23	20	18	WEDNESDAY
24	21	19	THURSDAY
25	22	20	FRIDAY
26	23	21	SATURDAY
27	24	22	SUNDAY
28	25	23	MONDAY
29	26	24	TUESDAY
30	27	25	WEDNESDAY
31	28	26	THURSDAY
	29	27	FRIDAY
	30	28	SATURDAY
		29	SUNDAY
		30	MONDAY
		31	TUESDAY

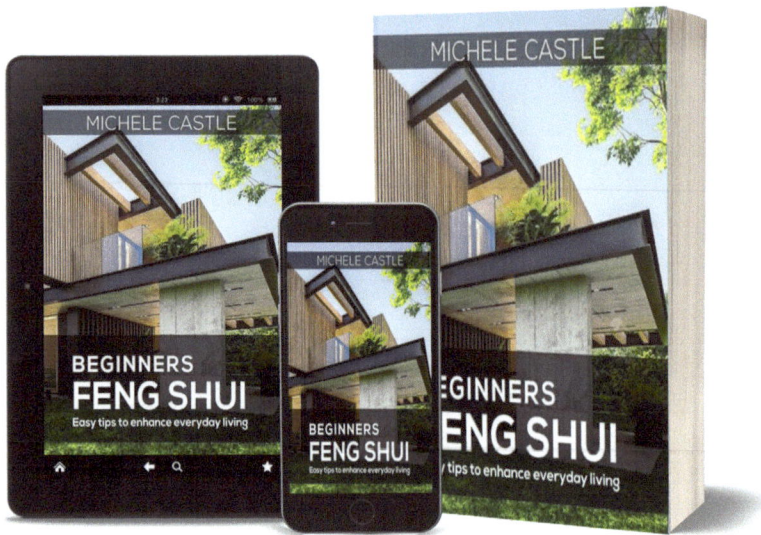

BEGINNERS FENG SHUI

'EASY TIPS TO ENHANCE EVERYDAY LIVING'

Feng Shui, the "art of placement and manipulation of energy".

Embark on a transformative journey into the ancient art of Feng Shui with "Beginners Feng Shui." This guide, meticulously crafted by Michele Castle, distils two decades of expertise into a comprehensive beginner's manual. Uncover the secrets of Chi energy flow and the art of placement to bring balance, harmony, and prosperity to your living space. Whether you're a novice eager to learn or seeking inspiration for your next home renovation, this book is the perfect companion. Delve into health, wealth, relationship, and career strategies through symbolism, placement techniques, and the use of colour. Elevate your understanding of Feng Shui with this insightful guide, ideal for learning enthusiasts and those looking to enhance their homes.

Available Audible, Ebook or hardcover https://amzn.to/3uCoMOU

DISCOVER THE POWER OF PERIOD 9 FENG SHUI AND CHINESE ASTROLOGY 2024 - 2044

Explore the captivating world of Feng Shui and Chinese Astrology with an Audible, Ebook or hardcover copy of "Period 9 Feng Shui and Chinese Astrology 2024 – 2044." Authored by Michele Castle, a dedicated expert in Feng Shui, this book unravels the mystique of Period 9, a twenty-year cycle from February 4, 2024, to February 3, 2044. Discover the transformative power of the Fire Element, fostering personal growth, creativity, and innovation. Delve into tailored Feng Shui techniques, aligning with the energies of Period 9, and envision your dreams becoming reality. Navigate cosmic influences with flying stars charts and dynamic period energy. Join a vibrant community of seekers ready to explore and connect on this enlightening journey. Michele Castle, a trailblazer in Feng Shui, invites you to unlock the secrets of Period 9 for a life-changing odyssey toward unprecedented success and prosperity. For inquiries or courses, contact

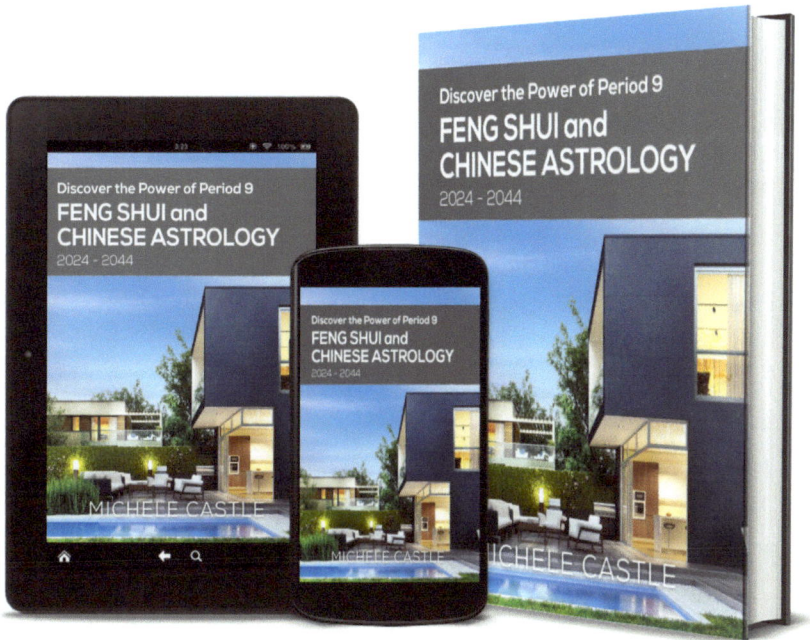

michele@completefengshui.com or visit www.completefengshui.com.

Available Audible, Ebook or hardcover https://amzn.to/47AyeRh

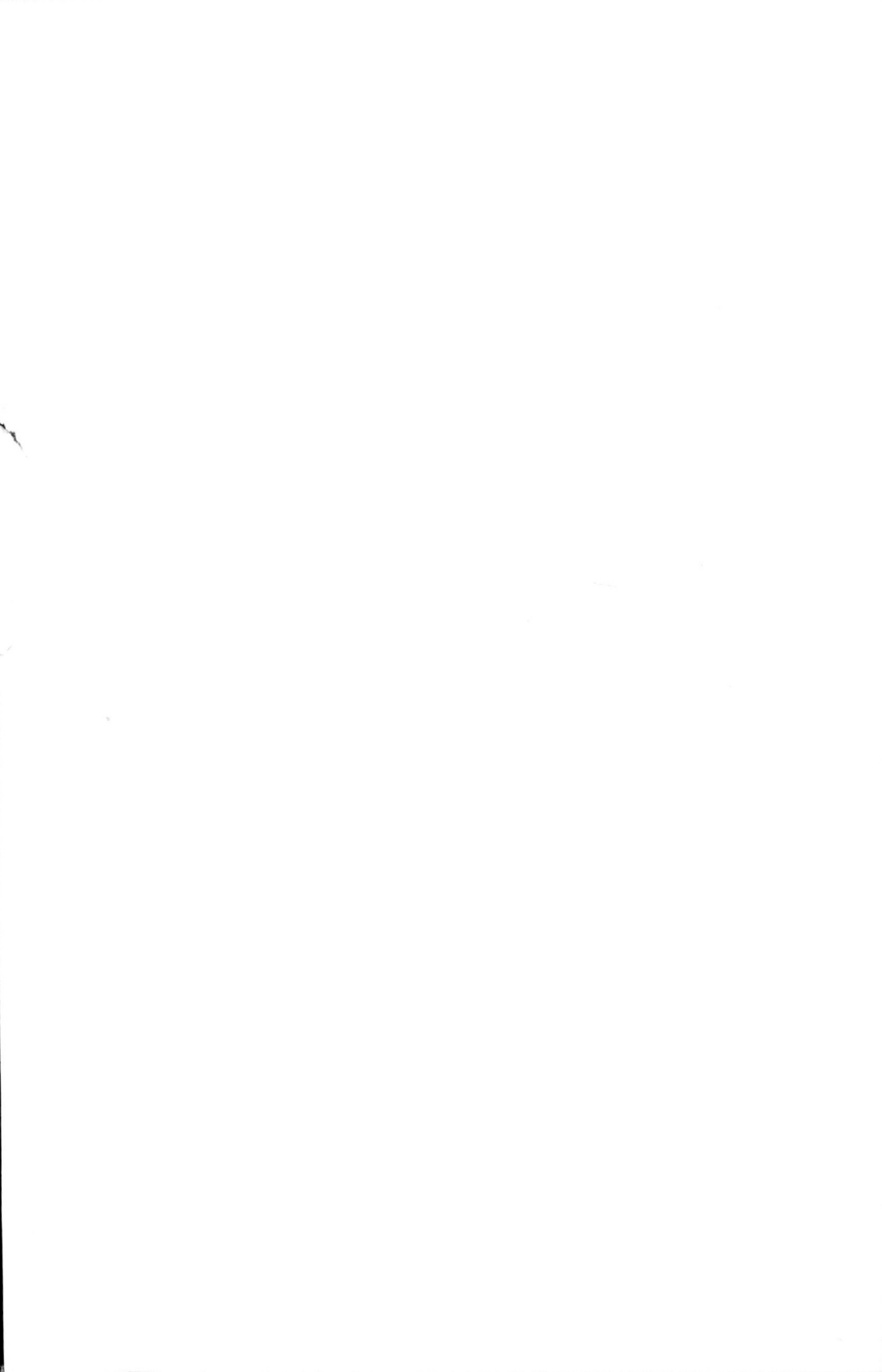

9 780645 909791